Meditations *on* Hope

Other books in the *Kaplan Voices: Nurses* series:

Reflections on Doctors: Nurses' Stories about
Physicians and Surgeons

Final Moments: Nurses' Stories about Death and Dying

Meditations *on* Hope

Nurses' Stories about Motivation and Inspiration

∾

Paula Sergi, BSN, MFA
Geraldine Gorman, RN, PhD
EDITORS

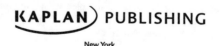

New York

© 2009 Kaplan, Inc.

Published by Kaplan Publishing, a division of Kaplan, Inc.
1 Liberty Plaza, 24th Floor
New York, NY 10006

Printed in the United States

Library of Congress Cataloging-in-Publication Data
Meditations on hope : nurses' stories about motivation and inspiration / Paula Sergi, Geraldine Gorman, editors.

  p. ; cm. -- (Kaplan voices)

 ISBN 978-1-4277-9824-4

 1. Nursing--Psychological aspects. 2. Hope. I. Sergi, Paula, 1952- II. Gorman, Geraldine. III. Series.
 [DNLM: 1. Nursing. 2. Nurse-Patient Relations--Personal Narratives.
 3. Nurse-Patient Relations. 4. Nurses--psychology--Personal Narratives. 5. Nurses--psychology. 6. Nursing--Personal Narratives. WY 87 M491 2009]
 RT86.M43 2008
 610.7301--dc22

                                    2008027141

10 9 8 7 6 5 4 3 2 1

ISBN-13: 978-1-4277-9824-4

Kaplan Publishing books are available at special quantity discounts to use for sales promotions, employee premiums, or educational purposes. Please email our Special Sales Department to order or for more information at kaplanpublishing@kaplan.com, or write to Kaplan Publishing, 1 Liberty Plaza, 24th Floor, New York, NY 10006.

Contents

Introduction

HOPE IS AN elusive promise—difficult to define, to contain, to make good on. No wonder Emily Dickinson imagined hope to be "the thing with feathers." Just when we think we have it caged, it soars from sight.

For nurses, hope presents a unique challenge. It wears different guises depending on one's area of practice, philosophical and spiritual mooring, and professional development. For the experienced practitioner, hope can germinate within the harshest of realities. In "Breaking Bad News," the revelation of an STD to a frightened young woman affords Cortney Davis the opportunity to encounter hope enmeshed with kindness as "a silent standing by—anything that might help steady the heart." Despite the stark, war-torn landscape of the Kosovar countryside, in "The Peaches," Nancy Leigh Harliss savored the promise of hope in women's laughter which transcended language barriers, sweet as the summer fruit that engendered it. Flight nurses encounter tragedy on a daily basis; small acknowledgments of their efforts offer the sustenance to continue. In Emily McGee's "Maybe It Was Enough," we see this firsthand.

Meditations on Hope presents nursing practice as a prism, refracting hope. These essays illustrate how nurses strive to nurture their own spirits of belief and optimism so that they can authentically share this with those for whom they care. Nurses struggle to convey hope to a patient with little chance of survival, as portrayed in "When the Patient Becomes the Teacher." As explored in "In Sickness and in Health," we learn they also struggle to support the loved ones who face inevitable loss. And yet as those two meditations so poignantly convey, it is often the nurse who draws renewal and regeneration from the therapeutic relationship.

How many chose this profession because of the illumination cast by other nurses? In "A Belated Thank-You," an anonymous ER nurse tending Karen Klein's lacerated knee lent the eight-year-old girl a magical courage, setting her firmly on her future professional path. "I am a nurse because of Karen," begins

Doris Urfer's account, "My Life of Hope." She writes of the pediatric practitioner whose relationship with the author's daughter brought hope to an otherwise sterile medical wasteland. Even as an 18-year-old student at the Grace General Hospital School of Nursing in 1967, Bonnie Jarvis-Lowe found inspiration in the stories of the women who came before her, all those "nurses feeding babies in the middle of the night by lamplight." As she recounts in "My Little Lamp," she carried a lamp forward with her as a reminder of what it means "to stand the test of time."

And of course, what nursing prism does not reflect both the radiance and shadows cast by the patients who share the journey? Laura Monahan learned an early lesson in the elusiveness of hope when, as a student nurse, she was first confronted by the stark reality of a patient's terminal diagnosis. In desperation, she sought her family's prayers for her patient's family; hope revealed itself to her in the "grace, courage, and tenacity" she witnessed in the nurses who persevere despite it all. The irascible Mr. Bunyan offered communion to Madeleine Mysko in the form of a sun-warmed tomato and, like the peaches of summer, she partook and found it "sweet indeed."

So welcome to these many faceted *Meditations on Hope*. St. Julian of Norwich, centuries past, promised that all shall be well, and all manner of things shall be well again. Whether on the chaotic medical surgical units, the adrenaline-drenched helicopter rides, or in the sanctified domiciles of families, nurses grasp hope to their breasts as a talisman and shield. It may absent itself for periods brief or extended, but with the faith of St. Julian, nurses scan the landscape for its return. In these tales arising from nursing practice, we witness the transfiguration of hope, sitting like a feathered thing, preening in the sun.

Meditations *on* Hope

Breaking Bad News

≈

Cortney Davis, MA, RNC, APRN

I PICK UP THE first chart. I'm about to flip it open to find out why this patient is here today when I see a note stuck on the front of the folder. *Positive for chlamydia* is scribbled in the secretary's handwriting. *Here for treatment.*

I'm tempted to put the chart back and let one of the residents deal with this patient, but it's high-risk-pregnancy day and we're already backed up. Anyway, I've been a nurse-practitioner in the women's clinic for more than 11 years and before that, a nurse in intensive care and on a cancer ward. Giving bad news is part of my job.

Reviewing the chart, I read that the patient, Ellen, is in the 14th week of her first pregnancy. Three days ago, she'd experienced burning with urination and vague pelvic pain. She'd come to the clinic, terrified that something was wrong with her pregnancy. The resident who saw her collected a urine culture to make sure Ellen didn't have an infection and did a pelvic exam, checking for simple infection, like yeast, and culturing for more serious infections. Yesterday, the nurse called and left a message on Ellen's phone: "Come into the clinic tomorrow. We have your test results." Looking at the chart, I find that everything came back negative except the cervical culture. Ellen has chlamydia, a sexually transmitted disease. Now I'm the one who must tell her.

Giving bad news to patients is a special talent, something no amount of education can teach. When I was in nursing school and later in nurse-practitioner training, there were no courses called "How to tell a patient she has cancer," "How to tell a father his child has died," or "How to tell a pregnant woman she has a sexually transmitted disease." Breaking bad news is an on-the-job skill learned only in the doing, in the holding of patients' hands, and in the simple comforting acts that suddenly erase the distance between patient and caregiver: the hug that keeps someone on her feet; the way we sometimes let patients see tears in our own eyes.

On the cancer ward, I perfected the arts of acknowledging the approach of death and staying with patients until death arrived. In intensive care, I learned to deliver bits of stunning information as if they were updates from some distant, unfamiliar city. Calling a newly admitted child's parent, I'd say, "Your son's been admitted to ICU." Then I'd wait a few seconds for the implication in my voice to travel the phone wires. Or I'd grip a woman by the shoulders and look into her face. "I was with him when he went," I'd say. "He didn't go alone."

When I came to the women's clinic, I thought joy would outweigh tragedy. Mostly, that's true. But bad news here is particularly difficult to deliver; it often involves new life, and it can pierce the soul. I've told mothers that their pregnancies won't survive. I've announced that my fingers have palpated the solitary, fixed breast nodule that could be cancer. More and more often, I have to tell young women that their bodies are infected with diseases they get only from making love. How, I wonder, will Ellen react to the news that she has chlamydia?

Some women nod and smile, unable to comprehend how they—who are faithful to their partners— could have a sexually transmitted disease. They look at me with such innocent bewilderment that I'm afraid for them. Then when they finally understand, they weep or become so angry that even the bland, beige clinic walls seem unable to contain their fury.

Other women blush and lower their eyes. These are the patients who have secrets to tell and, sometimes, they tell me. The brief affair. The man who they thought loved them more than their husbands. These women are dazed; they thought they were only following their hearts. When I say, "You'll have to notify all your partners," these women see themselves abandoned and alone. "How can I tell my husband?" they ask. I never have the right answer.

Most often, patients receiving bad news crumble before me. Their skin blanches. They lose their breath, as if punched in the stomach. It's difficult to watch their suffering. I've found it's best to give bad news over time, bit by bit, like you'd give a child small bites of food that are easier to swallow. Patients can only take in what they're ready to accept. Of course, bad news must be followed by a list of options, as if those might be the sips of water that help soothe the lump in the throat. If we can offer patients new tests, specialists to see, the possibility of cure, then we can also give them hope. After so many years in health care, I've learned that all we can really give our patients is what we would want for ourselves. We can listen without judging; we can accept that we are—after all—like our patients: stripped, raw, and vulnerable.

I take the chart and go into room four, where Ellen sits on the exam table. A man—I assume it's her partner—waits beside her on a chair. "Oh," I say to myself. "This will be twice as hard."

"Hi Ellen. I'm Cortney, a nurse-practitioner here in the clinic." I extend my hand to her, then face the man. "Hi," I say. "And you are. . . ?"

"Max," he answers.

"I got a message about test results," Ellen explains. "Is everything okay?" She rests one hand on her belly.

This exact moment—the uncertainty and possibility contained in the brief pause before I answer—is one of the things I dislike most about delivering bad news. Perhaps this is because I never plan what to say ahead of time, but wait until I can evaluate a patient's emotional reserve and then intuit how to proceed. Straightforward? With a maternal hug? Offhand and casual?

During this pause, I also feel guilty, as if I'm not simply a messenger but also somehow responsible for a patient's soon-to-be-visible anguish. I've learned that words are like stones. Tossed into the vast expanse of a patient's life, their impact causes shock waves. In ever-widening circles, everyone is affected. What

was to be a patient's future is wrenched into a different shape and becomes, eventually, the past she'd like
to forget. Sometimes, patients forever associate caregivers with the information we've delivered. I don't
want to cause pain. Like any nurse or doctor, I want
patients to like me.

A physician once told me that he "soft-pedals"
the news, making a dire situation sound not so awful.
He wants to spare patients pain, but I think evasive-
ness leads to confusion. I can't skirt the issues to avoid
hurting a patient's feelings. At the same time, I want
to be gentle. I know what it's like to have everything
changed by a single test result or one damning word.

Ellen, even before I speak, looks hollow, as if the
smallest blow could shatter her. Max looks anxious. I
picture them raising their individual shields against
anything that might alter their world.

"Ellen, I have your cervical culture results. Do
you want Max to be here when we discuss them?"

I sit down by the exam table so I'm close to Ellen.
After all, she is my patient. Part of me wants to say, "Tell
him to leave. You might want to hear this alone." But
there's another side of me, one I don't like, that wants to
say, "Let him stay. Let him be devastated too."

"Yes, I'd like him to stay," she says.

I've never met Ellen before, not an uncommon
occurrence in the clinic and in this era of managed

care. In some ways, I'm glad. Being the messenger can be more difficult when I have a long-term relationship with a patient I've come to care about. In other ways, sometimes it's easier when I've treated a patient over time. Then when I arrive with disastrous results in hand, she knows I'll support her, that her misfortune will become our common grief.

"Ellen, your culture came back positive for an infection called chlamydia."

"Oh God. Is that something that could hurt the baby?"

"Not if it's treated, and we've caught it in time. I'll give you an antibiotic to take right after we talk. Your baby's going to be fine. And Max?" I turn to him. "You'll have to see your doctor and get treated too. It's important that you refrain from intercourse until you've both taken medication."

Max opens and closes his hands. I notice he's not wearing a wedding ring.

"I don't understand," Ellen says. "How did I get this?"

"Chlamydia is a sexually transmitted disease. You get it from having sex with someone who has it."

"But I only have sex with my husband."

"You get this infection when you have intercourse with someone who is already infected."

If I have to, I'll say this over and over. Bad news has to be given in short, strong sentences. Otherwise, it's impossible to hear. Even when it involves the simplest absolutes—he's dead; she has cancer—bad news takes time to understand. I see Ellen struggling: if she only has sex with Max, she caught this infection from him. If she has sex with other men, this could have come from any one of them. Once a man or woman has this infection, they can spread it to every partner they have.

The room is uncomfortably quiet. My pulse quickens. I want to make everything better. I could say, "It's very common—more than four million cases of chlamydia occur annually in the United States," but that would be soft-pedaling, turning the attention away from Ellen's individual dilemma.

"I only have sex with Max." She looks at me as if I might shelter her from the image that, like a sudden eclipse, has darkened her imagination.

"Sexual intercourse is the only route of transmission." I place my hand on Ellen's knee. Tears fill her eyes and she purses her lips. When she goes to wipe her cheek, she begins to sob. I stand and put one arm around her, mindful of the newness of our relationship and the ambiguity of my role. I bring both the poison and the cure.

Max stands too. "I don't have any symptoms. I couldn't have given her anything."

"This infection might not cause any symptoms. That's why it's so difficult to detect."

"This means Max got it from someone else and gave it to me?" Ellen's face is blotchy.

"I don't know, Ellen. Chlamydia can be dormant in the body for months."

She speaks first. "We've been together three years," she says.

"Married for one," Max adds.

"Does that mean you've only been faithful to me for one?"

I don't interrupt.

"Tests can be wrong," Max says. He paces beside Ellen, who now holds both hands on her not-yet-enlarged belly, as if to cradle her fetus.

I say, "The type of test we use is rarely inaccurate." I'm accustomed to this back-and-forth rapid firing of questions. Such a debate always occurs as patients sort and assimilate the facts that accompany bad news. How did it happen? When did it happen? Are you sure? The last question patients ask—the one that I can never, ever answer—is why. Why did this happen? Patients think bad news might be easier to accept if only it came with some reason, some lesson, or someone to blame.

"We're having a baby," she says, half to me and half to Max. "How could you do this?"

"I didn't do anything," he says. "I could never do anything like that, and you know it. You know me."

I try to read his anger, then hers. Defensive? Honest? If I could ignore her embarrassment and his indignation, I might suppose they were the perfect couple. I never know which patients will someday become the recipients of bad news. You can't tell just by looking.

"I recently spoke to another couple with the same problem," I say. "They decided to trust each other—they both said they had no other partners—so they took their antibiotics and moved on. We have to treat this infection. But I know it's not as easy to heal the emotional effects."

In the grand list of bad news, some items are worse than others. I feel better when I can convince myself that bad news might also be the beginning of recovery, as I hope it will be for Ellen and Max. But in the end, grief is grief. It doesn't come neatly measured, and we can't compare one pain to another. There's nothing to be gained by telling a patient, "It could be worse." For Ellen and Max right now, this is grief enough.

I give Ellen four antibiotic tablets and watch as she takes them. I hand her a pamphlet about chlamydia. Max says, "Can't you treat me too?" and I tell him that this is a women's clinic. We don't treat men. He accepts this explanation but tips his head as if he hears something behind my words. Later, I'll replay our conversation. After all, I'm still trying to learn this technique, the best way to give bad news. Do I take sides? Even when I try not to, do I sometimes point a silent finger? Later, I'll wish I had a neat formula to follow. Then I'll think . . . no. Only we humans give and receive bad news. It must remain, therefore, a messy and imperfect skill.

In this case, I'll never know if the chlamydia test was falsely positive, if Ellen had another partner, or if it was Max who'd had a fling. One thing I know about bad news is that it often comes out of nowhere. Once it arrives, it never really goes away.

I shake their hands and say I hope I'll see them again. I ask Ellen to call me if she wants to talk or has any questions. When they walk out of the exam room and down the hall, Max takes Ellen's arm. She doesn't draw away.

We caregivers sometimes have allies when we give bad news—patients find information on the Internet, and there are support groups for every ailment. Nevertheless, the initial announcement of bad news is always a solitary event, shared by patient and caregiver. When I'm the caregiver, all I can do is try to bring kindness, as well as truth, to the encounter: a hand's brief pressure, a silent standing by—anything that might help steady the heart.

Julia
(or the Burden of
Bearing Witness)

~

Keynan Hobbs, MSN, RN

Julia came back to the unit today, where I work as a psychiatric nurse. The story that is passed among the staff is that this time she checked into a hotel in a manic state, bought almost $800 worth of food and crammed it into the kitchenette, and after a week caused a scene that brought the police.

I ask her how in the world she had spent $800 on groceries.

She says angrily, "They were staples!"

The attending and resident assigned to Julia decided to file for conservatorship for her because she has been in the hospital so often in a short amount of time.

She asks me, "Why can't I just go back and live in the house I'm paying for? That I own half of? That my family takes advantage of me to live in? I gave up a life of my own to buy that house!"

I ask her what she means about giving up a life of her own, but she doesn't respond. She's not keeping eye contact now, sitting with her hands folded in her lap, and starting to cry and rock back and forth. I think she is now somewhere far away from where this conversation started. She says, "My mother told me that house would always be mine!"

When Julia starts to talk about her mother, a bright red hue creeps up her neck and face until it overtakes her whole head. It is remarkable against her white hair. I give her chances to regain control on her own, then I do a grounding technique that brings her back to the present and the red tide slowly recedes until Julia is not happy, but at least isn't shouting, crying, and clenching her fists. She recounts to me how she was abused as a child. This isn't the first time she's told me about this, but it isn't any easier to hear than any of the other times.

I get her some medication. I used to avoid using medication to help her calm down, because it made me feel like a failure and because when it was offered, Julia would often say mockingly, "Oh sure, Julia, here's more medication, take it and shut up!" I went one shift with her insisting on only using verbal intervention; I really gave it my best. And it was good—but not good enough. It only put her on a roller-coaster ride of calm and rage: up and back down, up and back down, up and back down. Now when I give her the medication and she starts with, "Oh sure, here's more medication . . ." I just tell her that she isn't being fair.

Later, Julia wants help mailing her nursing license renewal. This has been an issue between us because she believes that I should see her as a peer, but I can't. I see her as too ill to practice, but she insists that she isn't. I can see and appreciate the nurse in her—in how she organizes our linen closet, in the volunteer activities that she tells me about, and in how she handles her medications—but I think I see it because she works so hard at showing it to all of us. She says it is evidence that she isn't sick—that everyone else around her is the problem, not her. But her actions are always tempered in some way by her mental illness: they may be nursing in spirit, but are no longer nursing in form. It is as though her judgment is simply gone, and that stands out as a significant reason for why I can't see her as a peer. I think that I will have to be clearer in my own mind about what a nurse is—and can be—before this conflict will be resolved.

IT IS TIME for a meeting with Julia's mother concerning the home they own together. When we enter the room, Julia sits across from her mother. I sit roughly between them at the end of the table, next to a social worker and a physician. Julia's mother is in her eighties and has a stone-faced affect. After brief introductions, the stage is set for some big news from Julia's mother: she states—slowly and matter-of-factly—that when the papers were drawn up to make Julia part owner of the home, the notary in attendance was a friend of the family and never intended to file the papers. Julia has never owned half of the house; telling her that she did own it, her mother says, was "to give you some sense of self-esteem."

Julia screams, "But I gave up my life to buy that house! I paid half of the down payment! I put on new windows, a new roof . . ."

Her mother denies that any of this happened, though she won't keep eye contact while doing it. "Any money that you might have paid into the home was rent as far as I'm concerned," she says.

Julia screams back at her about the years of abuse she endured.

"Julia, you are like a dog," her mother says, and she looks straight into Julia's eyes for this. "You are like a dog that has broken through thin ice and lots of people are all coming out to you . . . and we can either let you drown or hit you over the head and save you."

BACK IN JULIA'S room, she is still bright red, scream-ing, crying. She sits in a chair, hunched over and yell-ing and pounding her clenched fists into her thighs. As she yells, I think about starting a grounding exer-cise for her, but I don't. I think about getting medica-tion, but I don't. Instead I kneel down and I put my hand on hers, a boundary I ordinarily might not cross, but just for a moment I put my hand on hers and I witness her suffering. I'm stripped bare by what I've seen today, and all I have left to offer her is to bear witness. And as Julia begins to quiet, I'm pleased to find that a witness is, in fact, exactly what she needs to get through this moment and on to the next. Julia allowed us to connect enough to get through this moment together, and that leaves me with hope that healing is still possible.

As a psychiatric nurse, I am often privileged to see the most personal and private parts of a patient's life. I may be the only person they can talk to about something, because I may be the only person in their life that isn't part of its cause. The incredible risk that comes with this is taking the stories in—and having no way to let them back out again; then they become a burden. I have many techniques that I might apply to any situation, but two appear to be essential for me to ease suffering and make positive change when it matters most: the ability to take in another's suffering and the ability to let it back out again.

When the Patient Becomes the Teacher: A Lesson in Hope

~

Dorothy Consonery-Fairnot,
MSHA, RN, CCM, CLNC

HAVE YOU EVER thought about how suddenly your life can change? I am a workers' compensation nurse case manager. The most challenging case of my career came when I was assigned to work on a catastrophic case involving a 23-year-old male who received an electrical shock while working on a construction site. By the time I was assigned to the case, Jim had undergone several surgeries as a lifesaving measure, which resulted in the removal of half his body (a hemicorpectomy).

This case was transferred to me when Jim was three months post-injury. Upon arriving on the ICU burn unit, I was greeted by the ICU case manager, who discussed the case in full and gave me an opportunity to read Jim's extensive medical record. The evidence was clear that although Jim had survived an accidental electrocution, several surgeries, and infections, he was not out of the woods yet. His condition was listed as stable but critical. My initial responsibilities included assessing Jim's medical, psychological, and social needs and condensing them into a comprehensive short- and long-term treatment care plan with a goal of having him reach his maximum level of functioning. Having to establish a long-term treatment goal was quite challenging because of Jim's condition and because the medical survival rate for such patients was poor. Based on these factors, I realized that to make the greatest impact on this case, I would have to use aggressive case-management interventions to maximize Jim's chance of recovering from this devastating injury.

Upon entering Jim's ICU room, I was met by his father, a man of small stature with eyes that cried out for answers. He could not speak English, but I knew the questions he—as a parent—must have: Why my son? Will he live or will he die? Will he be an invalid for the remainder of his life? I gestured to him and tried my best to explain that I was there to help his son. The father's nod let me know that he understood that I was there to help. I knew then that all of my future visits would require a professional interpreter.

Jim lay motionless in bed but opened his eyes once; clearly he was medically sedated to allow his body to heal from the sheer physical shock of losing so much of his body mass. Imagine the impact of a multisystem body trauma: there are so many deficits that your body has to learn to compensate for that. It is no wonder that few survive this type of body-mass loss. But Jim was alive—and fighting.

Make no mistakes: his physicians were amazed that he was still alive, but they did not give me false hope. His chances of survival and full recovery were poor.

I visited Jim weekly while he was in ICU, and I spoke with the ICU case manager several times during the week. To everyone's amazement, Jim's medical condition was improving day by day. My patient survived ICU and spent another nine months in an inpatient rehabilitation center. He gained use of his left arm. His right (dominant) arm had to be amputated, disarticulated at the shoulder level. In total, Jim spent more than a year in a hospital setting being nursed and rehabbed back to a full medical recovery.

The numbers of major and minor surgeries he endured were countless—let's say more than 20, including several skin grafts.

Rehab taught Jim how to strengthen his left arm and how to make this his dominant arm. His upper body became very muscular and strong enough that he was able to use the overhead trapeze bar to pull himself up while in bed.

Remember, this young man now had half of his body; his surgery included a disarticulation at his hip level. He could not turn himself, but he learned how to roll over by himself. He was fitted with a thoracic bucket to fit into his wheelchair.

Jim surpassed all expectations and triumphed over every obstacle. Above all, he did it with such human dignity, becoming an example to all who worked on his multidisciplinary team. Jim had the courage, wisdom, and ability to see that self-pity meant defeat—and that wasn't a part of who he was.

As professionals, we were challenged by his decision not to accept sympathy: life had much more to offer him than sympathy. We were cautioned that Jim could become depressed. I remember one group session that included his psychologist, who reported that Jim was not showing signs of depression but that she wanted him to remain on the antidepressant medication. Depression could cause a major setback in his treatment. I was thankful that that day never arrived.

During his care on the rehab unit, Jim's psychologist found a church-affiliated hospital volunteer group that taught English to non-English-speaking patients. In one year, Jim went from uttering a few words in English to speaking and understanding the language very well. He learned how to paint landscapes; I have the two pictures that he gave me hanging in my office as a reminder that true courage can lead you to a greater place.

My goal was to transition him from a rehab facility into a handicapped home setting. I was faced with many challenges in my collaborations with everyone who was involved in his case, which included attorneys, adjusters, employers, and several physicians. I cannot stress how important it is to develop trusting relationships with all parties involved in your case, conveying the central message that you are a nurse advocating for the best medical care on behalf of your patient.

In the course of arranging for Jim's discharge home, I arranged for a handicapped van and for him to attend college to learn computer graphic art. What a joy it was to see him go to college. He was so excited and he talked and talked about the other students he met.

Jim was very fortunate in that he had a father and sister who relocated to this country to take care of him, which allowed him to remain in close proximity to the physicians who saved his life. Jim's family was truly a major support system, providing him with love and excellent home care. With a good family support system, even severely injured individuals have been known to increase their life span.

During the course of four years that I managed this case, I experienced so many emotions. I was taken to another spiritual level by my interactions with Jim. I had never seen such real hope, courage, dignity, humility, and strength—and it came from someone so young.

There was a bond between Jim and his physicians that I had never experienced in 25 years of nursing. I felt it when I was in their presence: they were a team who fought this fight together, and they won. I heard physician after physician tell my client's story: someone greater than us spared his life so that everyone who encounters him will see hope and love of life in action.

Is there a greater gift for humankind than this? Jim never lost hope, never became depressed or angry. Instead, he was an inspiration and a lesson in compassion and hope for all who had the privilege of treating him.

My Life of Hope:
One Nurse's Story

~

Doris I. Urfer, LPN

I AM A NURSE because of Karen. I am a nurse because every doctor and every specialist told me that my daughter Angie would die before she reached her first birthday. I am a nurse because hope helped me conquer the tests, the pain, and the trials that life has put me through. The story of my daughter's illness and recovery is one nurse's story of hope.

Forty-six years ago, on August 19, 1961, the weather was terrible in Havana. Rain was pouring down on our way to the airport. As we arrived, we were brought over to a glass-walled room to check in. It looked like a fish tank. This was the room all Cuban citizens had to pass through to travel outside the country. Officers took my ring and my necklace as collateral to ensure that I'd return, along with my family, once our government-issued travel visas expired. I didn't know it then, but I was leaving Cuba forever, in the company of my parents and sister, to a land I would come to love. I was only 17, very scared, and afraid to speak because, well, I didn't know English.

Life in Miami was difficult in the beginning. My father had to earn an income, so he left to work in the Dominican Republic with colleagues who had also fled the lost country we had called home. Meanwhile, I fell behind one year in high school because of the transition. My mother used her skills as a seamstress to work in what some people call a sweatshop, but what she always just considered to be her job. All this time, I was determined to do two things: learn English to the best of my ability and become a U.S. citizen. By 1970, I had done just that, although English is an ongoing struggle of adjectives, verb tenses, and my accent.

Three years later, I met Fred and became his wife. Fred—Bud as we all call him—made my life complete with his generosity, sense of humor, and comforting ways. Most of all, he inspires me with the love he has for his children. He is the love of my life.

Out of this wonderful marriage, we created two beautiful children—our firstborn, Freddy, and 22 months later, Angie. Angie was born the morning of Wednesday, April 18, 1979, with the blue sky in her eyes and the sunshine in her hair. She thrived until she was about three months old and then mysteriously developed a rash. I wasn't concerned at first, but the months passed and the rash persisted. After multiple trips to different doctors and specialists and numerous tests and biopsies, her pediatrician discovered Angie was born without an immune system. She could not fight infection or any disease because her bone marrow produced nonfunctioning white blood cells. Even a simple cold could kill her. Angie was diagnosed with severe combined immunodeficiency (SCIDs), an extremely rare and fatal disease.

It is estimated that 1 in 69,000 babies are born with SCIDs. Angie's prognosis was poor at best: most SCIDs babies don't survive past their first year. She was in serious trouble. By the time Angie was nine months old, Dr. Giusti, her Orlando-based pediatrician, told my husband and me that there was nothing more he could do for Angie in Florida. Our only option, he said, was a bone-marrow transplant.

We were given no promises. We were told that Angie's body could reject the bone marrow, leading to certain death. In addition, we were told that unless we found a 100 percent match to Angie's blood type, there was no chance whatsoever of a successful transplant. My husband only matched half, I only matched half, but Freddy, barely two years old, matched 100 percent. So on December 27, 1979, my husband, the children, and I departed Orlando to try to save Angie's life. Angie was admitted to Boston Children's Hospital Medical Center, the only location in the country where such a transplant could be performed.

Prior to the transplant, Angie was given medications to kill the cells that were attacking her. These medications caused her to lose her hair; the cartilage in her nose deteriorated from the multiple tubes that helped her breathe. The chemotherapy left her with the risk that, long-term, Angie would become sterile. But none of that mattered. Our only hope at that moment was for our daughter to survive. Angie received her transplant on January 17, 1980. It was only the eighth transplant of its kind in the United States.

Moving to Boston from Orlando was a shock to my system. We had no home, minimal health insurance, knew no one in the city, and the weather... let's just say it's not Florida. After the transplant, my husband returned to Florida with my son. I stayed in Boston, alone with my daughter for the next four months.

After the transplant, Angie had to live for four months in a glass-enclosed, germ-free room at the hospital. If this sounds familiar, it is. It's the same disease, same treatment, and same story as that of David Vetter, whose long fight with this disease was made into the television movie *The Boy in the Plastic Bubble*. Angie's bubble room had a crib and a rocking chair. The only people who could go inside her room were those who scrubbed for five minutes and wore gowns and gloves. The same rules applied to me. I only held and touched my daughter through latex gloves. I only looked in on her through a wall of plastic. I always knew that the experience would be a tough battle; I never imagined the isolation and despair I'd feel as Angie fought day after day.

I lived in the Ronald McDonald House for a month and later moved to a two-bedroom apartment closer to the hospital, which I shared with another couple whose daughter was ill. We supported each other as much as we could. We even went to Fenway together one day.

I wasn't all alone. The hospital staff was generous with me. And Angie had many wonderful nurses taking care of her. One particular nurse made a big difference in my life: Karen. She was always there to listen to me when I was worried, giving me hope when the doctors told me there was no change in Angie's condition. Her kindness and the way she cared for her patients, especially my daughter, were priceless.

I spent each day in the hospital from 7 AM to 11 PM. If Karen and the other nurses had to work late, I'd run back to the apartment and make a big bowl of spaghetti so they'd have some dinner. When Karen worked nights, she'd walk me home. We'd chat about Angie, about ourselves, and about life. I always hoped that the doctors would give me good news about Angie, but it was Karen who kept me going. Karen is a remarkable person, a wonderful nurse, and a true friend. Karen's impact on my daughter and myself has stayed with me, long after our days in Boston.

Finally the big day arrived—and it happened to be Easter. What a wonderful feeling! Freddy's T cells were working in Angie's body. The transplant was working. Then, finally, I was able to enter Angie's room with just a mask, no gown or gloves. I cut the ribbon at the doorway. I was so afraid to contaminate her that the nurse had to push me inside. The minute Angie saw me, she extended her little arms so I could pick her up from the crib and, as I did, she pulled the mask off my face. It was the start of getting to know my daughter again after those four long months. Angie was just the third person to survive SCIDs in the United States. We came home for good on April 24, 1980.

Seeing how my daughter was treated by all the staff was wonderful. All the nurses were so kind, but seeing Karen's relationship with Angie, and how much she cared for her well-being, has always stayed with me. It's why I am who I am.

I AM LUCKY to be where I am. I love my job. I love being a nurse. The minute I'm in the hospital, I can't wait to check my patients to make sure they are okay. There are multiple people with multiple needs that I can solve. I have patients who don't speak English, and I can see the fear and doubt in their eyes. They're in a giant fish tank. But I speak with them, put them at ease and at peace. It makes a big difference. I can take care of my patients on so many different levels, just as Karen and the other nurses took care of Angie.

Nurses aren't just about checking vitals and following a doctor's orders. We are so much more. We are that bowl of spaghetti. We are the walk to an apartment at 11 PM when you don't know if you'll see your daughter alive again. Nurses are a shoulder and a hug and a light when everything looks bleak.

Hope is a nurse. It has helped me obtain everything I've wanted. My daughter and I are living proof of that. Angie is now 29 years old, married, and even though the doctors told her she probably could not have children, she has two beautiful sons. I am a proud grandmother and in my 25th year of nursing. We are so proud of our son Freddy, of the doctors, and of the nurses for allowing Angie to become the miracle of life that she is.

A Belated Thank-You

~

Karen Klein, RN

Has a total stranger ever suddenly come into your life, had a profound impact, then gone out of your life just as quickly, leaving you permanently changed? Someone did just that in my life and left a deep, positive impression. She is someone who will never know the effect she had on my life and consequently, on the lives of thousands of other people. This is a story about one nurse, one day, many years ago.

In August 1970, four days before my eighth birthday, I cut my knee when I fell off the top of our pool ladder and landed on the ground. The first thing I remembered was my sister, who was nine and very squeamish, looking down at my knee, then running to get my mother, all the while screaming hysterically, something to the effect of "Karen fell and her knee meat is hanging out!"

I looked down at my knee where the skin had been so cleanly sliced by the edge of the aluminum ladder. Just below my kneecap was a laceration a full inch in length and a good half-inch deep. Because the slice was so quick and clean, there was no blood. "Cool," I thought, inspecting the wound closer. "That's a little bit of what I look like inside."

My mother appeared upset when she looked at the cut. Her hands started to shake and she told my sister to get the next-door neighbor, a friend of hers, who ended up driving us to the local hospital (what was then Mid-Island Hospital in Bethpage, New York). When we got there, the nurse took me into an examining room and laid me down on the table. I was a little bit nervous, looking up at the giant overhead operating light.

The fact that this was going to end up being painful finally dawned on me. I started to cry. My mother told me it was okay, she was right there, but she looked pale and worried as she stood over by the corner of the room. I was scared but the nurse gave me a tissue and began talking to me as she inspected and cleaned my knee with antiseptic—assuring me it would just feel cold.

"So, how old are you?" she asked among other questions, like what grade I was in and what school I went to and if I liked my teacher.

"I'll be eight in four days," I told her. Then, to garner more sympathy, I added, "I was supposed to have a pool party. I have one every year."

I figured I wouldn't be able to now because I kept asking my mother in the car on the way to the hospital and she said she didn't think so, but part of me hoped the nurse would say I'd still be able to. My hopes were quickly dashed.

"Looks like you'll have to plan something else special this year, right, Mom?"

My mother, her face drained of all blood, managed a weak smile. The nurse, who had finished cleaning my knee, gave her a seat over in the corner.

Then the doctor came into the room. He turned on the big, round overhead lamp and focused it on my knee. Then he put on rubber gloves. It was doom time to me. I must have looked scared. The nurse looked right at me and said, "I have a magic trick so that you won't feel any pain in your knee when the doctor sews it up. Here's how it works: When I say *go*, close your eyes, cover your ears, and hum. The doctor is going to pinch your knee for a few seconds, so it might sting like a bad bee. Have you ever been stung by a bee?" I told her that I had. "Well, it'll feel just like that—a big, bad bee. But if you just close your eyes, cover your ears, and hum until the doctor stops pinching you, you won't feel a thing after that, I promise."

"But after he pinches it, doesn't he still have to sew it back together?" I asked, still a little skeptical—and scared.

"Yes he will," she answered, "But if you close your eyes when I tell you to, cover your ears, and hum until he stops pinching your knee, you won't feel anything when he stitches it. That's the magic!" she added with enthusiasm.

She spoke so confidently that I couldn't help but trust this total stranger. I hoped what she said would be true and sure enough, after doing what she said, I felt nothing after the initial pinch. The magic had worked!

I was lying flat on my back and I could see the doctor's hand coming up with the needle and thread, but I couldn't see what he was doing. He asked me if I felt anything, and I assured him that the nurse's magic had worked.

"Are you sewing my knee together now?" I asked.

"Yes he is," the nurse answered.

"Can I watch?" I asked her.

My mother, who was still in the corner looking away, let out a groan.

"Sure!" the nurse said enthusiastically. The doctor stopped momentarily, the nurse sat me up by adjusting the table, and I watched the remainder of the procedure. I was fascinated. And it was completely painless!

"Mom, I think we have a future nurse on our hands," the nurse told my mother, who managed another weak smile.

On the way home from the hospital, I confidently informed my mother that when I grew up, I was going to be a nurse so that I could help other people just the way that nurse had helped me. She took me at my word too. When recounting the story to others of how I watched the doctor suture my knee while she sat in the corner, fighting nausea, my mother would call me her "future nurse." She even wrote it in my sixth-grade graduation autograph book: *To my future nurse . . .*

The years went by. When I was a senior in high school, it came time to decide what college I would attend and what I wanted to do for the rest of my life. This is a tremendous and confusing decision for most 17-year-olds. For me it happened in one moment. My guidance counselor had informed me that in addition to several other scholarships for which I was eligible— owing to my high grade point average—there was a health career scholarship that I could apply for and receive, but only if I chose a profession in the health care field.

It was then that it struck me. I had always said I wanted to be a nurse when I was younger. Of course! I remembered so clearly, as I still do today, the nurse who had helped me as a child. Yes, I was suddenly sure that was what I wanted to do.

Four years later, after graduating with my BSN, I took the state boards and became an RN. I've never regretted it. It remains the one decision that has most affected my life.

Thirty-five years after my brief encounter with that nurse, I still marvel at how profoundly she affected the direction of my life. I often think, "What if I had been younger and unable to appreciate this nurse's intervention?" or "What if it had been a different nurse with a different bedside manner?" or "What if the same nurse had been overloaded with patients and did not have the time to give the attention she gave to me?" There are so many what-ifs, but one thing is certain: had I not encountered this particular nurse on this particular day, my life would have turned out very differently.

So this is my belated thank-you to an unknown nurse who never knew the influence she had on my life. It is a thank-you as well from the thousands of patients who, in turn, I have had the opportunity to help during my own 26-year nursing career.

My Patient, My Hope

~

Mary Jeanne Creamer, BSN

I ONCE EXPERIENCED A moment in my nursing career that was not only a monumental triumph in my patient's life, but it was also the moment in which I finally found closure for a rather difficult chapter in my own life. The experience gave me the ability and courage to forgive and move on.

I was out jogging one afternoon and was hit by a speeding car. Everything went blank: I had suffered a severe head injury. My prognosis was extremely critical. The doctors could not tell my husband in what condition he would get his wife back if and when she left the hospital. I was 37 years old and had just had my wonderful son, Daniel Ryan, not even a year before.

My recovery was long, painful, and slow. I spent days in and out of physical, speech, or occupational therapy. I looked like a monster. I had had a craniotomy and lost hearing in my right ear. Half my face was completely paralyzed. I couldn't take a step without falling. And the pain. . . My eye would not close due to the antiseizure medication. Sometimes my two sons were afraid at just the sight of me. Even thinking about it all now is overwhelming.

THE YEARS PASSED. My progress was slow. I would get so angry. How can I ever be a good nurse again? Why did this happen? Why did I have to run that day? I often wondered if I would ever be able to return to work as a registered nurse. My physical recovery was one hurdle; my professional rehabilitation was another.

I eventually did get back to working as a nurse with constant tenacity and help from all the wonderful nurses I worked with. My life was finally beginning to resemble the life I had lost three long years earlier. When I returned to work, I made the decision to never discuss my story with my patients, although I am sure some of them wondered what had happened to me because of my appearance.

Several years passed and I was doing well. I was healing physically and emotionally and—oddly enough—I was working on a brain injury unit. So it happened that I met a young man who was a patient on the unit. He was 22 years old and was the victim of a drunk-driving motor-vehicle accident. His head injury was severe. It ran chills up my spine to see a person who had had a craniotomy just as I had. He lost his left eye and there was a very good chance that he would lose his right leg. Days turned into weeks. I was his nurse every day. Finally, when I saw cognitive improvement, I decided to tell my patient my own story.

It was the first time I ever really spoke about it, and he never stopped asking me questions. When I came on shift, his face would light up. I believe I became his inspiration.

Eventually, my patient was discharged. I think of him so often. Like myself, his entire life had been put on hold. He became engaged six months before his accident, and he had just finished a graduate program to teach science.

Some time afterward, I was working and a young man I did not recognize approached me. Then, of course—I knew. He, like myself, had finally pulled through his nightmare. He now walked with a cane and had a patch over his eye, but I knew his strength and courage could not be measured by his appearance.

He was getting married in two months and had gotten a teaching job!

Ours was a shared bond of spiritual accomplishment. We both persevered and triumphed over insurmountable odds.

An Unforgettable Experience

~

Rashida J. Merchant,

BScN, RN, RM

As a routine in the ob-gyn unit, shift-over used to be face-to-face from last shift team leader to next shift team leader. One day about four months after I graduated from a nursing diploma program, I was the team leader in the morning shift.

"Thank God we are finishing off. It was a hectic night shift for all of us," said Yasmeen, the night shift team leader. Yasmeen was reporting with a long face during shift-over in the conference room.

As we proceeded, Yasmeen reported on a patient, Mrs. Danyal, a primigravid 32-year-old, who was shifted from labor and delivery at around 3 AM. Mrs. Danyal delivered a baby boy (weighing 3.8 kg) through spontaneous vaginal delivery. Yasmeen went on to report that Mrs. Danyal had a difficult night—which was tough on everyone. On and off, Mrs. Danyal kept pressing the call bell for assistance in passing urine. She had been taken to the toilet or given a bedpan several times but did not pass urine. Yasmeen reported that Mrs. Danyal's vital signs were within normal range. Her last reading was taken at 6 AM, and it was normal.

I visited the patient as soon as I finished with the shift-over at around 8 AM. Mrs. Danyal was in noticeable discomfort and was moaning with pain. I asked her how she was feeling and if she needed to use the restroom. She refused to go but asked for the bedpan.

Out of habit, I had my fingers on her radial pulse while talking to her. Within a few seconds, I realized that I could not feel her pulse. I asked a midwife to help Mrs. Danyal with the bedpan and rushed to get a manual blood pressure (BP) apparatus. (We did not have a wall-mounted BP apparatus at our institution.) I checked her BP but could not find it. I immediately asked another nursing colleague to check her pulse and BP. Meanwhile, I sent out a rush call to the on-call resident. My colleague confirmed that there was no pulse or BP.

The on-call resident, Dr. Maria, and primary consultant, Dr. Alisha, came running from labor and delivery. They assessed the patient and passed on Foley's catheter. Dr. Alisha examined Mrs. Danyal and found that there was a huge hematoma on the posterior wall of her vagina.

Dr. Alisha had asked for a BP reading at 7 AM. But because that was time for shift-over and Mrs. Danyal had been considered a stable patient, her BP reading was not checked at 7 AM. Dr. Alisha was highly disappointed and actually shouted at us for not keeping the patient's hourly BP record.

Mrs. Danyal was immediately sent to the main operating room to drain the hematoma. Approximately 1,000 cc of blood were drained from the hematoma. She received two pack cells and was kept under close observation for the next eight hours. Luckily, Mrs. Danyal recovered fast and was discharged within four days of her delivery.

Mrs. Danyal provided me and my colleagues with a priceless lesson that will last a lifetime: never assume that patients are just being difficult. They have reasons for being uneasy.

A Daily Dose of Hope

~

Jessica Gallinaro, RN

Hope shines through in the most delicate of moments, and usually when you need it the most. As a nurse, I am always looking for the light at the end of the tunnel or that patient that makes me remember why I decided to become a nurse in the first place. I have to say, it sometimes takes weeks for those moments to present themselves, but when they do I take them as a direct gift from God.

I have been a nurse for three and a half years, and I have gained an enormous sense of pride and accomplishment from the profession. Nursing school provided me with the skills and techniques I needed to be successful, but nothing could have prepared me for the sense of self-worth and importance I would feel once I started working. This didn't come right away, and some days it's hard to feel it, but I know it's there. It's there in the thank-yous I get from patients and in the kind words they write and send to the unit. It's there in the smiling faces of people who are sometimes too sick to get out of bed, and it's there when those people actually walk off the unit upon discharge.

With all the meaningful and uplifting moments that occur in the hospital, there are times when a nurse wants to throw in the towel and head for the hills. My motto is, "Put a smile on your face, even when you're crying on the inside." As nurses, we have to find our "happy place" multiple times throughout the shift in order to keep our sanity. We may understand that sick people don't always treat others with the respect that they normally would and that family members of these sick people tend to raise their voices a little quicker than they normally would, but that doesn't make it any easier on us. I will never forget one such patient and her two daughters, to whom I am grateful for teaching me to truly listen to what family members have to say because they are usually right. Unfortunately, I had to learn in an environment that caused severe headaches, anxiety, and produced a shadow, which was not my own.

THIS PARTICULAR PATIENT was on my unit for a few weeks, and this is unusual, since the normal length of stay is 24 to 48 hours. I was not the nurse for this patient for the first week she was there, but I quickly learned of her story and that of her two daughters. It was difficult not to. They were constantly at the nurses' station yelling and banging their fists on the counter demanding to speak with this doctor and that doctor. In any normal circumstance, this would be alarming and a cause for concern, but in this circumstance, the behavior was particularly unwarranted. I knew that their mother was very ill, but we were doing everything we could for her and her illness was not a free pass for causing an uproar.

Finally, the day came when I had this patient on my assignment. When I realized this, my heart started to beat a little faster and I began to panic. I was convinced the two daughters were going to eat me alive. Before entering the patient's room, I made sure I knew every last thing about her, about all her medications and about her plan for the day. I wanted to have an answer for any question that was thrown at me. Luckily, the first issue was easily resolvable. They wanted their mother to get a certain pill at exactly a certain time. In the nursing world, medications can be given an hour before or an hour after they are ordered, but if they wanted a med given on the dot, I was going to do that. The two daughters quickly realized that I was on their side, and I was only concerned with the health and safety of their mother. Eventually, I won them over. It took a few hours and a lot of paging doctors, but it happened. They were tough, but after a few days of caring for their mother, I realized that they were just scared; scared of losing her, and I couldn't hold that against them.

I CARED FOR this patient a few more times after that and even when I wasn't her nurse, I would stop in to say hello. The patient made a great recovery, and she became stronger and stronger. She was actually taking steps by the time she left us. Compared with not even being able to roll over in bed, this was pretty amazing. In the end, the daughters were grateful for the care that their mother had received. Watching them leave the hospital with a healthy mother was one of those gifts I was talking about, but the even bigger gift came a few weeks later.

About a month had passed when the patient and her daughters made their first visit. They were glowing with pride from all the obstacles their mother had overcome. We welcomed them with hugs and kisses. Once a patient is on a unit for a long time, they become like a family member. It was very fulfilling to see the patient with her lipstick on and her hair and nails done, bragging about how far she could walk now. The family was very appreciative of all our hard work and dedication to their mother. They were at ease on the unit, which was a complete change from when their mother was a patient. Every once in a while, we receive a letter from one of the daughters giving us an update on her mother. And every time I read one of them, I am hopeful that I will be able to touch another person's life as I have touched hers.

Maybe It Was Enough

~

Emily J. McGee, RN

"AERO MED FLIGHT crew, you have a confirmed flight request. Watership County scene."

I responded over my portable radio to acknowledge that I heard the tones and was headed out to prepare for the flight.

I grinned seeing the look on Ben's face. He was an army medic before he became a critical-care nurse, and today he was doing a ride-along with my flight crew. This is what he had hoped to be a part of.

He followed me to the hanger as I packed the blood cooler. It is standard for us to fly with six units of packed red blood cells. It has meant the difference between life and death for countless patients whom our flight team has transported. I hoped the blood wouldn't be needed.

I quickly reviewed with Ben the role he would play on the flight. We walked toward the aircraft, feeling the heat waft through the hangar. It was still warm for a fall day.

The flight physician, Steve, repeated for us what little report we were given from the scene, "Single patient ATV accident with head injuries."

Ben glanced at me, then at Steve. "That's all the information you usually get?"

I smiled. Steve responded, "We are lucky if we get that much!"

I made sure Ben was strapped in and that the internal radios worked. This was going to be a lengthy flight. We were responding to a recreational area quite far up north. Quite literally, there was nothing for miles.

Other than Ben's nervous leg bounce and his alternating between smiling at me and staring out the window, the flight went without a hitch. Our pilot set us down on the middle of the rural road, on the marked, improvised landing zone, like a butterfly with sore feet. The pilots like to say that: "We just drive the bus." But they play an awe-inspiring role in what we do.

I took one more look at the medical compartment of the aircraft. The stretcher was set up just how I like it. Steve was gripping our trauma bag. I had already given Ben the portable pulse oximetry monitor. It is always better to give someone who is nervous something to do—a lesson I learned a long time ago.

The engines stopped and the blades came to a halt. As we walked the 200 yards to the back of the waiting ambulance, the local fire chief met us to give a quick rundown on what had happened in the 30 minutes we were airborne.

"This lady went around a really bad curve and was thrown from her four-wheeler," he said. "She hit her head really hard. She hasn't been conscious for us at all."

My heart went to my boots. This wasn't good.

"How long was she out there before the medics arrived?" Steve asked.

The fire chief gave the last answer I wanted to hear: "About half an hour or so. She was way back in the woods."

Steve went in the side door of the ambulance to get to the patient's head as quickly as possible. Ben, who was attached to me at the hip, went with me through the back doors. He took the patient's right side as I took the left.

The medics were working furiously at establishing IV lines and attempting to use a bag valve mask to ensure the patient was getting enough oxygen. Her breathing was irregular and ominous.

Steve asked questions, attempting to piece together what happened. I began my assessment, keeping an eye on Ben. His focus was startling for someone who hadn't spent much time in the field. The medic nearest to me said that they hadn't been able to get a measurable blood pressure. My heart sank further. This lady was going to die and there wasn't much we were going to be able to do about it.

"I got an 18 gauge in her right AC!" a medic said.

"Nice!" I congratulated the medic—who was as relieved as I was. Getting successful IV access in a patient with an unreadable blood pressure is beyond difficult. It is life-sustaining. Emergency treatment for a trauma patient with low blood pressure is massive amounts of IV fluids and blood. Without at least one good IV, the patient could die.

We turned the flow of her IV fluids wide open, the medic instinctively squeezing the bag to get the fluid into her veins more quickly.

Ben elbowed me, gesturing to the pulse oximetry monitor as I quickly pulled out the IV medications I would need to paralyze and sedate the patient enough to insert a breathing tube. It was either not giving us an accurate reading or her oxygen levels were dangerously low. Her jaw was partially clenched, soft where it shouldn't have been. It was obviously broken.

Steve's eyes met mine as I lined up my RSI (rapid sequence induction) drug syringes. During long flights when I think I am going to need them, I pre-draw my medications and label them. It allows for less error in the midst of the controlled chaos. I was once again relieved I had done so.

"Hey, what is this lady's first name?" I asked over the noise. This question, as always, brings the noise down. It causes a slight group hesitation, reminding everyone that this isn't just another horrible accident. This is someone's loved one.

"Terri. Her name is Terri!" piped up one of the firefighters who was enlisted to help.

"Terri, we are going to put a tube in your lungs to help you breathe. We are also going to give you some medicine to help with the pain," Steve told her, although she was unable to respond.

"Steve, are you ready?" I asked.

This is the moment in which we as a nurse-physician team have to stop to ensure we are both prepared to take total responsibility for our patient's life. We were about to completely paralyze her, which meant she would die if we didn't do everything right. Her ability to breathe was about to be completely gone.

I glanced up through the haze of voices and the many hands and bodies doing everything possible to save this woman's life, and I saw a man. He was looking through the doorway separating the ambulance's patient compartment from the driver's compartment. I wasn't sure who he was or why he was looking at me with a blank stare. That brief interaction triggered something in my mind, but I shrugged it off, refocusing on what we were about to do.

I handed Ben the first medication syringe because the only IV was closest to him. On our flights, we allow those who ride along to practice at their level of licensure and comfort level. In Ben's case, trusting his skills was easy. Not only was he an amazing nurse, he happened to be my best friend. For me, it was like having an extension of myself.

"Lidocaine is in!" Ben said over the noise.

I glanced at my watch to mark the time. Steve continued to ventilate the patient as best he could, given her facial injuries.

Ben continued with the pain and sedation medications, which were carefully chosen to guard her low blood pressure. He verbalized each medication before he pushed it into the IV line, hesitating long enough for anyone not yet ready to stop the process. I knew he was nervous, but to the ground crew he sounded like he had been doing this for years.

"Steve, are you ready for the paralytic?" I asked.

"Yup. Go ahead," he answered.

Ben waited for my nod and pushed it. We all watched as her body visibly relaxed.

This was the point of no return and Steve didn't disappoint. The breathing tube went in easily. There was no audible air over her stomach, and lung sounds heard in every part of her chest.

As the medics helped Steve secure the breathing tube, I continued with the rest of my physical assessment. Bruises over her ribs and flank began to show. Her pelvis and legs were stable.

The medics ensured that the straps on the backboard and her head, which were securing her spine in alignment, were in place. Nothing else could be done. Her life now depended on rapid transport to a trauma center.

I jumped out of the ambulance. The fire chief handed me the helmet my patient had been wearing. It was of the full-face variety, the inside saturated with blood. The outside sustained frighteningly little damage. Whatever hit her went through the opening where she was wearing goggles.

As the medics began to off-load the stretcher, I asked the chief if she had anyone with her.

"Yeah, this guy was with her," he said.

I looked up at a man's face and at that instant realized that he was the man who was watching me from the front of the ambulance: her husband.

Ben, Steve, and the medics began walking down the paved road toward the aircraft. I told Terri's husband to walk with me. I started asking about pertinent medical history and allergies, trying to be as confident and soothing as possible. His flat affect and difficulty in answering simple questions concerned me.

I stopped in the middle of the rural road and softly grabbed the man by his shoulders. "Look at my eyes."

I needed him to focus on me, not on his wife, who was being wheeled to the aircraft on an ambulance stretcher. I stood close and forced myself to focus entirely on him. He snapped out of his panic and looked at me.

"We are going to do everything we can for her," I said. "I need you to focus on driving safely to the hospital. Your wife is going to need you."

His stoicism cracked. "Please," he pleaded, "you have to save my wife. She is all I have."

His words hit like a hammer. "Sir, we will do the very best we can," I told him.

Choking back a sob, he entreated, "Treat her like she is your own. Like she is your family."

I blurted out, "I promised my father once that I would do just that."

I gave both of his shoulders a squeeze and asked for his cell phone number so I could call when we arrived in the trauma bay. It was going to be a three- to four-hour drive before he would see his wife again. He nodded and I released him into the care of the fire chief. My mind focused back on the tasks at hand.

Terri was just about loaded into the aircraft, Ben was strapped in, and my equipment was accounted for. Steve was working one-handed, breathing for her with the other.

In the loading rush, between doing four different things at once, I leaned over to Ben and gave him a quick peck on the cheek. I knew I didn't have to explain why to him. He knew it was my way of acknowledging our friendship, the fragility of life— and what he meant to me.

Instinctively . . . airway, breathing. This basic component of any emergency medical scenario flitted through my mind.

Her airway was controlled with the breathing tube; air was passing in and out appropriately. We were able to monitor the amount of oxygen and watch the electrical waves of her heart leave waves across the screen.

Circulation. She needed blood. She needed more IV fluid. I still couldn't get a blood pressure. Air goes in and out, blood goes round and round, all bleeding stops eventually.

I strapped into my seat, hands busy with medications. I handed Ben a unit of blood and the appropriate tubing. I then slid the IV fluid into a bag designed to apply constant pressure, allowing me to get the lifesaving fluid into her veins more quickly.

Her rapid heart rate worried me almost as much as the lack of blood pressure.

The next time I picked up my head, we were 2,000 feet above the ground, flying as fast as possible. The pilots always know when to push the aircraft.

The 30-minute flight was both too long and not long enough. It's always a relief to be on the pad, just minutes from an entire team trained to save the unsalvageable. The duration of the flight is also a race to get as much done as possible before we land.

I handed Ben yet another set of IV tubing, IV fluid, and blood. The last thing I needed to do was put in a second IV. I ran on instinct, trying not to think about how I was going to manage it with the shake of the aircraft, the time pressure, and the fact that we were still getting such horrible blood pressure readings, if any.

"Flight com, show us on final," the pilot transmitted over the radio. We had about two minutes before landing.

There was no time for a tourniquet, which helps plump up veins, so I did a blind stick in her wrist. The aircraft was shaking as is normal during landing. A flash of blood filled the distal part of the catheter assembly. I advanced the catheter, putting pressure above the site while simultaneously removing the safety needle. Blood dripped out the end. I knew I was in, but held my breath. Without speaking, Ben handed me the connection end of the IV tubing. As soon as it was screwed in place, he opened the line. More lifesaving fluid began dripping into her vein.

Tape in place, aircraft parked on the roof, I transferred pressure bags to the stretcher as the aircraft engines spun down.

About ten minutes prior, Steve had given the radio report. The entire trauma team awaited us.

I recycled the blood pressure cuff: 85/40, our first measurable blood pressure reading of the flight. If only it were enough. Maybe it was enough. Please let it be enough.

A THANK-YOU ARRIVED in my email inbox a few months later:

I remember watching the helicopter take off and feeling like that was the last time I would see my wife alive again. By taking the time to call and let me know you arrived at the hospital and Terri was still alive, you gave me the strength to get through the remainder of my long ride there. The specialists told me they had done all they could and to "prepare myself." It is by the grace of God that she made it, and I thank Him for providing the skill of the people on scene like yourself.

It was enough. It is why I fly.

Cravings

~

Tilda Shalof, RN, BSCN

WE CRAVED FOOD for thought, as well as spiritual sustenance, physical rest, and time away from this demanding work. We had to take good care of ourselves if we wanted to do the work of taking good care of others. Sure, we were tired and hungry, but it wasn't sleep or food that we needed.

What we craved was spiritual regeneration and emotional nourishment in order to do this work properly and cope with its emotional demands. We desperately needed to fill up on whatever the commodity was that became so rapidly depleted within each of us from constantly attending to others' limitless needs. We needed replenishment of the spirit so that we could go on amid all the sadness and despair that surrounded us and not be downed or drowned by it.

We had thrived on the emotional support and understanding that we had received from our former manager, Rosemary, who was a nurse to the core. We felt gratified when our patients improved or when we managed to lessen their suffering or when we were thanked or even acknowledged. But more than anything, what quelled our longings, restored our souls, and satiated our appetites was the emotional and spiritual nurturance that we received from each other. It was what sustained us.

We debriefed one another after an upsetting encounter with a patient. We shared the horrors of wounds we had seen, patients' discomforts that we could not ameliorate, and heartbreaking tragedies we had witnessed. Who else but another nurse would understand how such things felt? It was from understanding that we derived the strength we needed to go forward.

We took care of each other. We shared secrets, the intimate details of our lives with one another. We understood one another. The work we did made us open up in this way. In fact, I believe that this closeness was the very thing that fortified us to do such emotionally demanding work.

But I was beginning to worry about the long-term effects of our constant exposure to suffering. At times I saw that it deadened us in certain ways and made us hypersensitive in other ways. More and more I saw that nurses were suffering. Nurses needed hope to go on.

"Who can keep it up for so long and remain caring all the time?" Frances asked with a huge sigh.

I looked at her. "If *you* can't keep it up, who can?" I said. "You always say how much you love nursing."

"The passion that drives me to do this work is the very thing that's going to make me leave it in the end," she answered wearily.

Somehow, of all of us, it was Frances who managed to forge a good relationship with the Lawrence family. One day they left a box of Belgian chocolates and a note at the nursing station:

Thank you to all of the staff caring for Irving. And a very special thank-you to Frances (she knows what for).
—Brenda Lawrence

I asked Frances what she had done to deserve that special mention.

"All I did was tell her, 'You do what you believe is right for your husband. Don't worry what the doctors and nurses say. After all, you and your son know him best.' That's all."

I marveled at the degree to which she controlled herself.

There were many times when we felt empty, bereft, overwhelmed by the demands—the emotional ones much more that the physical ones—of being nurses. Sometimes it seemed that the work asked too much of us, not only as nurses, but also as human beings.

We were not supposed to have our own needs. Yes, we were tired and hungry, but who cared? Certainly not the patients, who were mostly unconscious and totally dependent on us. Definitely not the families, who expected complete devotion from us and seemed to resent it when we took a break or even when we got up to leave at the end of a 12-hour shift, and they had to become accustomed to the style and idiosyncrasies of a new nurse.

"Are you back tomorrow?" families often asked as your shift was winding down.

You try to discern from their voice or the expression on their faces if they are relieved or disappointed when you say, "No. It's my day off." You know sometimes they ask for you specifically, and sometimes they ask specifically *not* for you, and you try not to care one way or the other.

It wasn't Florence Nightingale they wanted. The real Florence Nightingale was a hard-nosed battle-ax, a military micromanager, and a slave driver. What they wanted was a sweet, altruistic, loving version of Mother Teresa. So few of us could measure up.

Flying by the Seat of My Scrub Pants

~

Angela Posey-Arnold, RN, BSN

Anxious anticipation filled me as I arrived a little early for my interview. I had been working for years as an RN in quality assurance within home health care. I rarely got to see a patient, and I missed the hands-on nursing. But the expectation of possibilities for the job for which I was interviewing was exciting. It was for the position of assistant director of nursing in a long-term care facility.

I never thought I would like working in a nursing home because of all the horror stories I had heard. I took the job because I thought it would be a stepping-stone to a job with the state. I knew I would want to change the world if I worked in long-term care. I got the job and got my chance.

I was hired at 10 AM in the morning on January 4, 1994. I remember the exact time because I had gone home to eat lunch only to get a call at 1 PM from the administrator asking me if I could go ahead and start work that same day.

I thought to myself, "This is a little odd. Why would he want me to work today? I haven't even started orientation."

I put on my scrubs and went back to the facility. The administrator seemed extremely nervous and told me that all I had to do was to be present in the facility for four hours. So that is what I did. He asked me to make rounds and get to know the staff and residents. Then he left. Little did I realize I was actually in charge. I was flying by the seat of my scrub pants. Oh, how green I was. If I knew then what I know now, I would have had the sense to be terrified. As it was, I didn't know enough to be scared.

The facility had just lost every administrative RN they had, from DON to nursing supervisor. They were all gone. I was the only RN they had. I know I should have probably run for the hills, but somehow I knew this was where I was supposed to be. I went back the next day and began to learn what was really going on.

There was overwhelming evidence that the nursing department was hopeless. The administrator spent all his time in his office with the door closed and his phone on "do not disturb." At the same time they hired me, they also hired Elizabeth as the director of nursing. She was scared to death and had no idea what to do. She couldn't teach me what she didn't know herself.

Staffing was terrible. Nursing care was worse. Many of the residents were in restraints; there were a horrible number of cases of weight loss, pressure sores, medication errors, odors, and residents being neglected. It was a nightmare for two weeks.

I went home every day exhausted; all I could do was pray. Because of my faith in God, I knew that he didn't like the way his children were being treated and he wanted change too. I also knew that I could only make changes with his help.

The staff walked around in a state of despair. They were so unhappy. Some of the nurses were just bad nurses, lazy and mean. They did not want to change and they resented my every effort. They knew I was about to turn their comfortable little world of laziness into one of work. Some were not willing to change and worked against me constantly.

The residents were unhappy. The families were unhappy too, and they were looking to me to change it. The facility was in trouble, but I had hope that things could change.

I did not know federal or state regulations even existed, but I did know good nursing care. I started to try to change things one resident at a time. I did have a nurse consultant from corporate who was available for me if I had questions. He was supposed to come and orient me soon.

I had been there for two weeks, flying around by my proverbial britches, when a very frantic nursing secretary summoned me to the front office. There in the lobby stood four women and two men. The administrator had gone somewhere without leaving a number for me to reach him. I quickly learned that these six very serious looking people were from the state. They were there to survey the facility.

The DON had gone to lunch, so I told the surveyors that I had been there for two weeks and I was in charge.

I called corporate and my consultant said, "Just do what they ask. I'll be there in four hours."

The surveyors remained in the facility for four days. Corporate came in like the cavalry, and my administrator spent a great deal of time in his office. I think he was crying. When he wasn't in his office, he was just standing around looking really stupid.

Elizabeth and I worked with the surveyors. Frankly, I was glad to see them. I was glad that they were there. For the first time, I had hope that things were definitely going to change. I had a feeling that a positive outcome was possible even when the evidence appeared to be to the contrary. We sure were getting a lot of attention from corporate, and that was exactly what we needed.

For the exit interview, when the surveyors had finished and were ready to leave, administration was called into conference—with some very angry surveyors. The evidence was overwhelming that the facility was in terrible trouble. They had written 38 serious deficiencies, most of them in nursing and dietary. In 1994, the problems were based on a scale and these all were level-A deficiencies, which meant that the residents were in immediate jeopardy. It meant that there was evidence of actual harm. The surveyors told us that we had 35 days to turn this all around.

They would be back in 35 days, and if they did not see drastic changes, the doors would be locked and the residents would be removed. I praised God. It was a blessing. This is exactly what I had prayed for: help. I had prayed for help and help had arrived.

The administrator was fired and a new administrator arrived the next day. The DON walked out without notice and I was offered the job. After I met with the new administrator, I decided to take the job. She and I were like two peas in a pod. We were on the same page, and we both knew that with God's help we could do this. We could affect change together. That hope immediately bonded and sustained us.

I was assigned a nurse consultant who stayed with me for the 35-day period. She was wonderful and taught me so much. The difficulties seemed to be impossible, but when we tackled them together, one by one, we began to foster change.

The nursing-care issues were never going to be fixed until we changed the heart of the staff. They had lost hope a long time ago. We knew that instilling hope in them was the only way to change the care they were giving. For years they had been left on their own. They had no leadership. They were like neglected children.

Most of them wanted to change; some of them did not. We slowly discovered who wanted change and who didn't. It was difficult to fire someone who had been there for 25 years, but it had to be done. We only had to fire a few new nurses. The others had good hearts and looked forward to the facility being better.

Within a week, the expectation that change was occurring created optimism in the staff. They began to anticipate that together as a team, we could make the changes needed to keep the facility open—and to keep the patients healthy and happy. For the first time in many years, it seemed possible to them that what they desired for the facility was likely to happen.

As time progressed and positive changes were made, there was a new feeling in the facility. The staff was happy and it showed. The residents started to feel that we really cared about them, and they began to hold up their heads and smile. The families realized that we were serious about changing the care that the residents received. All this newfound hope led to positive attitudes and perseverance from the staff.

Our administrative team was consistently professional and executed the plans for change. We needed to prove to the staff, residents, and families that their hope was not in vain. As a team, we realized that we were free to change the circumstances and that together we could do it.

Every couple of days, we would post a large banner at the time clock. We used acronyms for *hope*. Each one instilled a positive attitude in the staff. It was a trickle-down effect. The more positive the staff became, the better care the residents received.

Some of the acronyms came to us from staff team members:

- Harnessing Our Power to Excel
- Heart Outreach—Positive End
- Healing Our Patients' Environment
- Have Only Positive Expectations
- Hearts Offering Professional Excellence
- Help One Person Excel
- Hats Off for Professional Excellence

Thirty-five days quickly passed. The state surveyors came back ready to shut us down. I have no idea of what they were going to do with 153 elderly or otherwise debilitated residents, but they were prepared to do what they needed to do.

They surveyed as we watched with anticipation. We had done everything we could possibly do to improve the care in 35 days. Now all we could do was sit back and watch. We had nothing to hide and told the staff to be courteous and honest with the surveyors.

The results were astonishing. Some of our residents had gained weight and no one had lost any, pressure ulcers were healing, and we had no new in-house acquired wounds. We had safely reduced the use of restraints, and we had programs in place to continue to improve quality of care. The odor was gone. The enhanced quality of care had taken care of that problem at the source.

The day came for the exit interview with the surveyors. We held our breath as they cited us with several level-B deficiencies, mostly picky physical plant stuff. There were no level-A deficiencies, and the ones that we had before were lifted. They were not going to close the doors.

Surveyors never compliment. They are there to find problems, not to pat you on the back. But before they left, they told us they knew the facility had changed the minute they walked in the door. They said it was amazing how the atmosphere had changed.

The surveyors just could not leave without writing a deficiency on something. They actually got under the outside Dumpster with a toothbrush and wrote us up because our Dumpsters were dirty.

Oh, they always kept a close eye on us and visited often. But five years and many surveys later, the nursing department earned a deficiency-free survey. They could not find one problem—testimony to excellent quality of care.

Hope had conquered! We had a huge party for every shift. The residents, families, and staff celebrated every victory together. We could not have done it without doing it as a team that really cared. We had evolved into a compassionate nursing department that took pride in the care we provided.

I thanked God because I knew it was by his hand that hope prevailed in a very ominous situation.

Angelic Nudge

~

Patricia Holloran, RN

I WORK IN A substance-abuse facility on the fifth floor: detox. When report was just about to begin, there was a phone call from the ER in the adjacent hospital. The crisis worker at the other end stated that a patient was psychiatrically cleared, ready to return. I had no idea what she was talking about.

"Let me ask the night nurse about this since I just got here and haven't received report yet," I said. I put her on hold and asked the night nurse about the status of this patient.

Justin was a 19-year-old heroin addict who was admitted two days ago. He had been relatively stable until the evening before, when he admitted that he had been planning on hanging himself before his mother had brought him in. He had the rope and was ready. Justin became very agitated and suicidal on the evening shift and said that he wanted to overdose and kill himself. The staff called 911 and off to the ER he went, along with an interagency form detailing the risk he was to himself. The counselor called the ER and highly recommended that the patient be admitted to the hospital's behavioral health unit.

I continued the conversation with the crisis worker, who said that Justin was not suicidal. I asked them to fax the documentation to us and, if they were sure he was safe, to send him back. Shortly after that, we received a call from Justin's mother asking if she could visit with him briefly. Usually we don't allow visitors during detox, but the situation merited a visit by this very worried mom.

During our daily team meeting, the discharge planner stated that there was a good chance that Justin would be accepted to a facility that had a new in-patient adolescent unit designed for patients just like him. But Justin had at least one more day of detox to complete before he could be admitted to that facility. The counselor agreed to have an impromptu family session to set this up and to just see how he was faring.

By the time we were back to the nurses' station, Justin had returned, and the tech was taking his vital signs. He looked dejected and angry. His mother arrived shortly thereafter, and they both went into the counseling office with the counselor.

About an hour later, I checked in with the director of nursing. I told her about Justin and our plan for him. I then went to the nurses' station to find the counselor, the tech, and Justin's mother all talking to him. His expression was sad and angry. It was obvious that he was becoming agitated. He stated that he wanted to discharge against medical advice. He wanted his mother to take him home. To her credit, she refused to let him come home until he had received all the recommended treatment.

I asked Justin what he was going to do when he got home, since he was already feeling so sick and depressed.

"I'm gonna f—ing kill myself!" he yelled back to me.

"Justin, are you serious?"

"No, you f—ing bitch. I'm kidding!" he sarcastically shouted back.

Justin was crying, moaning, and begging to be allowed to go home. He was changing his mind every few seconds about staying or going. His face was beet-red and his breathing was labored.

We still had not received the fax from the ER to tell us what treatments, interventions, or medications that Justin had received. Even so, we offered Justin his detox meds, but he refused. Our unit is a low level of care. We do not have the ability to care for unstable psychiatric or suicidal patients, which is why it was so important to have Justin evaluated in the ER to determine the risk he may have been himself and to determine the safest level of care for him.

I was very alarmed, but tried to remain calm. The counselor was talking to him in calming tones, and the tech was also providing reassuring comments. We knew that we had to keep Justin safe—and in view at all times. I had no doubt that he would try to harm himself if he were left alone.

Suddenly, Justin opened the door and bolted across the hall for the elevator. The counselor ran after him and was able to get him back into the nurses' station. At the same time, I called 911 to have this suicidal young man taken to the ER for the second time in less than 24 hours.

I wondered how Justin was ever deemed to be safe by the crisis worker at the ER—especially since he seemed like he was even worse upon his return. The evening shift had sent the interagency form outlining his behavior from the night before, and then there were the counselor's recommendations. The ER had never faxed to us the information that I requested about anything they may have done for Justin during the night, such as any medication given or any psychiatric evaluation conducted.

I called the ER to inform them that Justin would be returning in a suicidal and agitated state and that we expected the ambulance momentarily. The crisis worker responded with a statement that left me speechless: "Well, this morning we contracted him for safety and he signed it, promising not to kill himself, and he said he wouldn't and then we let him walk back."

If I could have reached through the phone and strangled her, I think I would have, but my response was, "We sent you a suicidal patient, with documentation to back that up, and you believed *him*? You felt that he needed a behavioral contract for his own safety, then you let him *walk over here this morning*? What was going to be your follow-up? That he was safe and honoring his contract? Can you please fax the ER chart to us?" And I hung up.

Justin was out by the elevator, pacing. He was surrounded by two counselors, the director of nursing, and myself. The other patients were fully aware that Justin was not doing well, and they were also nervous. The staff tried to keep them away as much as possible.

About 20 minutes passed, but the ambulance had yet to show up to take Justin back to the ER. We were trying to keep him in front of the elevator so that the EMTs could take over as soon as they arrived.

I told Justin's mother what we had to do, and she seemed alarmed that we thought he was "that bad," but relieved that he was being taken care of. We did not tell Justin.

We were still waiting for the ambulance. Precious time was passing, and we were having increasing difficulty containing this troubled and frantic young man.

Justin went back into the nurses' station and sat down. I went back in with him. Through a wall of windows, I could see the counselors and his mother waiting by the elevator for the EMTs to come help take Justin to the ER.

Still no ambulance. Justin was very quiet, which was unnerving since he had just been begging to go home . . . just to go home.

It was such a muggy day for February. The windows were open about three inches and the air conditioners were on. The DNS office did not have the three-inch stop on her window. Suddenly, Justin jumped up from the chair, hugged his mother, and bolted down the hall. The counselor and his mother were racing after him, and I was close behind.

I will never forget the indescribable, gut-wrenching, terror-filled scream from Justin's mother. I knew that he jumped even before I ran into the room. Everything happened in milliseconds. I ran into the room to the dazed and unbelieving expressions of the counselor and Justin's mother in front of an empty window that framed the gray sky. The counselor and his mother turned and ran toward the stairs. I looked down. I saw Justin flat on his back in the low hedges about 20 feet out and about five feet to the left. He was alive. He should have been directly below us on the concrete. . . .

I RAN DOWN the steps to him. He was moaning, trying to get up. Unbeknownst to me, our tech was taking a smoke break about four feet from where Justin landed. She responded immediately, keeping Justin calm and immobile.

The ambulance arrived—28 minutes after we called them. They transported Justin to a trauma center: he had broken his back and both of his ankles. Thankfully, he was not paralyzed. An angel must have nudged Justin that far over into the hedges.

Maybe now Justin will get the care that he needs. In a strange way, he saved his own life.

In Sickness and in Health

~

Amanda Goodwin

ONE SPRING DAY, I went to my hospital ready for just another day in the field I love. One of my assignments was a patient with multiple sclerosis, an exceptionally devastating disease. As MS progresses over the years, it slowly injures a person's nerves, impairing physical functions: walking, talking, simple movements, cognitive functions, sensation, sometimes even breathing. It is indiscriminating and ruthless. One statistic I read said that 15 percent of all MS patient deaths were caused by suicide.

When I first went in to see my patient, I was unsure of what to expect because MS cases can vary so greatly. I was surprised to see a beautiful woman, a little older than my mother, lying in bed with a well-dressed man in the chair by her side. I could tell by his face that he was friendly but had a defensive guard up to protect his vulnerable wife. They both smiled and seemed genuinely happy to meet me, instructing me to call them by their first names, Jim and Ellie, instead of Mr. and Mrs. Carson. Ellie was quick to explain, "I'm not Mrs. Carson. Mrs. Carson is my mother-in-law!"

I soon found out that Ellie's particular disease process caused her to be bed- or chair-ridden, and she only had control of one of her arms. She could not even sit forward on her own for me to listen to her lungs. She asked Jim to do most of her moving and lifting, and I could tell she had deep trust in him. I asked how long they had been together, and they were excited to explain that they had been married for 37 years. As Ellie later shared with me, she met Jim at a friend's wedding not too long after she was diagnosed with MS. They were both in college at the time and quickly fell in love. Jim obviously saw beyond her health difficulties and found her beautiful soul. The rest was like a fairy tale—only in this one, the villains were severe chronic illness and the grim expectation of the always-progressing path of MS.

Throughout the day, I couldn't help but to really observe this couple. Their relationship was truly captivating.

Ellie couldn't do much completely independently. She could speak well with the exception of sometimes forgetting a word or a date. Cognitively, she functioned pretty well, and we had many conversations. Ellie could move one arm, but she was otherwise nearly paralyzed. She and her husband seemed to be affluent, and from what I gathered, Jim was able to take care of Ellie most of the time, which I'm sure was a large factor in strengthening their close relationship.

I have never witnessed such a deep trust as I did with this couple. Ellie literally depended on her husband for everything, and I could tell he was far beyond just being used to it: he was good at it too. Jim knew every single medication his wife took and didn't even have to think twice about the dosages and number of pills. During morning med pass, when he thought I gave her one pill too few, Jim questioned me and had me go over the drugs all over again. (It ended up that she was scheduled to get the remaining pill at bedtime.) He could describe in great detail all of Ellie's previous hospitalizations and illnesses. He knew exactly how she liked things, and he knew exactly how to hold her to carry her to the chair or the bathroom. He could sense her needs even before she expressed them, and he knew how to handle or perform every single component of not only her physical health, but her emotional well-being. The way Jim explained things to me, I knew he had lived most of his life trying to keep his wife as happy and healthy as possible. When she hurt, I sensed pain in his eyes. When she was frustrated with herself, I could see his disappointment. His questions to me were so well conceived that I knew he was determined to really understand the answers so he could digest the information that his wife could not.

Theirs was a seamless relationship. He instinctively knew when to pick up where her capabilities no longer reached. He knew her limits like a science, and he let her do for herself what she could. For the rest, he jumped in like her savior and communicated what she could not express and assisted where her strength failed. There were no gaps in this love. There was no doubt that they were as one person. None at all. They shared feelings, fears, knowledge, and most importantly, such a primitive, deep trust.

I learned a lot from Jim and Ellie. For me, the learning was just more personal, a little deeper. I myself have been dealing with a chronic illness since I was five years old, and now that I am engaged to be married, my disease has become even more real. My fiancé is wonderful and his love is strong enough to see me beyond my illness, but I still struggle with so many thoughts, questions, and fears.

I'm so thankful for Jim and Ellie. A single day with them renewed my hope and helped me to see how strong love can be. I wonder how Ellie told her husband-to-be about her illness. I wonder what thoughts ran through their minds. What were they afraid of? What obstacles did they have to work through? Was she embarrassed at first for him to see her at her worst? I'm sure Jim and Ellie spent a lot of time getting to know each other, and Jim undoubtedly worked very hard to be to his wife what he is today.

Nevertheless, as I know all too well, fear clings to illness. I wonder how afraid Ellie is. I wonder if Jim knows just how much he means to his wife, or is he just focused on taking care of her and keeping her comfortable day-to-day? I wonder if Jonathan and I will mesh like that when we're their age. Will he be such a seamless part of me that he can feel what I feel, know what I know, and fix me before I even know I'm broken? Will he know just how essential he is to my happiness, safety, and well-being? Will he know selflessness is never taken for granted? Will he know he is really loved even when my strength fails me?

Love, as I saw that one spring day, is strong, humble, and desperate. If you stop to ponder it, love's beauty will take your breath away.

The Peaches

≈

Nancy Leigh Harless, NP

We have to laugh, because laughter,
we already know, is the first evidence
of freedom.

—Rosario-Castellnos

"OH! NANCY'S PEACHES are delicious!"
Nurse Dijetare said, giving her long black hair a toss,
her dark eyes uncharacteristically bright as she drew
the words out salaciously and set off a wave of laughter
among the quarantined medical team.

I worked in a medical project as part of a large
postwar recovery effort in the Balkans. My job was
to train Muslim Albanian nurses and doctors in the
basics of prenatal care. Scattered about the Kosovar

countryside were little *ambulantas*—stark, tiny clinics with only the most basic equipment.

Throughout the scorching summer, while hot winds howled like mournful hounds through the half-opened windows, we worked together side by side to bring prenatal care into remote areas where the concept of seeing a clinician throughout a pregnancy was as foreign to the village women as this plainspoken American who had just offered up her peaches.

The previous week, one of the doctors came down with rubella and exposed the entire unvaccinated Kosovar medical team to the disease. Immunizations were just one of the many things unavailable to Albanian people under the harsh Serbian rule prior to the war.

The doctor was sent home to recover, the others put in isolation for three weeks to assure they too did not break out in the red spots that could be so damaging to a growing fetus. Now, instead of spending their days in the villages providing care, they were confined to the office.

The brighter side of the quarantine was that at least it gave us time to spend on training. It seemed odd that an American nurse-practitioner would be teaching doctors; however, the alternative education system they had trained under was sorely lacking. Medical training for the Albanian Muslim doctors had been thwarted by political unrest during the past

20 years. When the Serbian Orthodox took power, they forced all Muslims out of government jobs and schools. The Albanians developed a separate, underground, parallel system of both medical education and health-care provision from their Serbian counterparts. They did the best they could under difficult circumstances; however, the young doctors who were educated in this system had large gaps in their training. Prenatal care, for example, was not addressed. But the fact that medical school was taught at all—literally out of homes and garages—was a shining tribute to the strength of spirit, resilience, and tenacity of these wonderful people.

But now time and funding were running out. We had only four months left to complete their training.

WE SAT ON hard plastic chairs, crowded around a small picnic table that served as our training center. It was uncomfortable, especially in the afternoon when the hot sun baked through the curtainless window and the sirocco-like winds blew in like an efficient central air system gone awry, blasting hot air into the room. I invited the women to the house I lived in next door to the office. The heavy gold brocade curtains were tightly drawn to block some of the day's heat. Surely we'd be more comfortable lounging in the living room than sticking to the hot plastic seats in the sweltering office.

"Get comfortable. I'll get us something to eat," I said as I led the medical team into the foyer and kicked off my shoes.

Each of the women removed their shoes and began to find a place on one of the long couches at both ends of the long, narrow living room. The nurses, Dijetare and Bedrije, sat on one couch; the doctors, Drita and Mirvete, sat on the other. Nurse Hamide sat quietly on the floor.

Although we had worked together only a few weeks, each of the women had shared with me at least part of their personal horror story of war. I was moved by how deep their need to talk about it was—their need to be heard. Without prompting, their sad stories spilled out, usually with tears, but sometimes dry-eyed and detached as if talking about something that had happened to a stranger a long time ago.

Except for Dr. Drita, who was a little older, all the women were in their late twenties or early thirties. They were just children when the Serbians took control of their country and their lives. All of the women carried the invisible weight of depression. It showed in their eyes and in the way they carried themselves, moving lethargically, in slow motion, as if only sheer will made them go about their activities of daily living.

Dijetare, a beautiful young woman in her late twenties, had thick, long, coal black hair she wore loose around her shoulders. She rarely smiled, and when she did, it was a tight, forced effort, like a model made to hold a pose too long. Dijetare's large, brown eyes held a hard history. Her hurt began with her father's death 20 years ago. A writer with unpopular political views, he was beaten and left in the forest with both hands severed. Dijetare was only eight years old.

At 22, Bedrije was the youngest of the women. Her blonde hair and blue eyes contrasted with Dijetare's dark, exotic beauty. Bedrije's cheeks dimpled when she spoke, especially when she spoke to the handsome young Conti, one of the young men who served as both driver and guard for the medical team. Bedrije was married—a loveless relationship—arranged early by parents concerned over her free spirit. She rarely mentioned her husband to the other women. Conti, on the other hand, came up often in conversations.

Hamide sat on the green shag carpet, legs crossed in yoga position under her dark gathered skirt. She sat quietly, not speaking, hands folded in her lap, brown eyes cast down. It was easy to overlook Hamide in a group. She was experienced at being invisible. Her father had died when she was 12. Her mother married soon after, but because children are considered their father's property, Hamide was sent to live with her paternal grandparents, a stern, serious couple that practiced the older and stricter Muslim ways.

"They are not . . . um . . . modern Muslims," Hamide told me earlier in the week as we practiced conversational English. "They were . . . disciplined. They allowed my mother . . . only little . . . visits to me."

Dr. Drita sank down on the far end of one of the long brocade couches with a heavy sigh and turned her head away from Dr. Mirvete, sitting in the middle of the couch. Dr. Drita had a port-wine birthmark on the right side of her face; she usually turned it away whenever she spoke. Her face was further disfigured by a flaccid drooping at the left edge of her mouth that caused spittle to gather and roll down her chin if not wiped often with the large white handkerchief she carried in her pocket. Dr. Drita was only in her mid-forties, but she looked at least 20 years older. Life and circumstance had not been kind to her. Her husband, also a doctor, was killed when they cared for Albanian resistance soldiers. Dr. Drita's life was spared, but she wore unspeakable scars just the same. She went about her work quietly, talking only when necessary. She rarely smiled; however, when she did, her entire face opened up. She had an incredible depth of spirit. When she spoke of her losses, it was usually in terms of how losing their father affected her children, a son, age 13, and a daughter, 11.

Dr. Mirvete was a large-boned woman with solemn, dark eyes and short, black hair. She translated for Hamide and Drita, who spoke less English than the others. She explained I was getting us something to eat. Mirvete often took a leading role with the group; she particularly liked to tell the younger nurses what they should do.

She was instructing Bedrije to "go help Nancy in the kitchen," when I walked through the doorway from the kitchen carrying a tray of fresh fruits and cheese. At the market the day before, I was amazed at the variety of fresh fruits and vegetables, as well as other things laid out on tables under red and blue tarp tents. There had been everything from fresh, plump, red-skinned ripe tomatoes to piles of dull yellow chicken's feet bleeding from their severed ankles. I could have purchased a knockoff Rolex watch or a live turkey, but instead left the market with a bag filled with only vegetables and fruits. What I was most excited about were the peaches—wonderful ripe, luscious peaches that hadn't been available on earlier market days.

I offered the tray to the nurses and doctors and said, "You've just got to try my peaches. They are delicious!"

My remark caused an uproar among the women. It began with only Bedrije snickering and nudging Dijetare in the ribs. Dijetare began to giggle, and then the entire group of women sitting on both couches began to laugh. Nurse Bedrije and Dr. Mirvete both spoke English very well. They kept repeating, "Try my peaches. Try my peaches. They are delicious," and laughing until tears rolled down their checks.

Nurse Dijetare translated for Hamide and Drita, who didn't understand at first; however, once translated, they too began howling in laughter.

"What? What did I say?" I asked as I laughed with them. I could tell from the sort of laughter it was and from the tone of their voices as they chattered among themselves in Albanian that I had made some sort of faux pas. The other women continued to howl and exchange remarks about "Nancy's delicious peaches." It felt good to see the smiles on their dark faces—faces that were usually held in tight masks. Their dark, sad eyes had all viewed scenes no one should ever have to see. I'd been with them for a few weeks and rarely saw them smile. The only other time I had heard their laughter was when we were frightened by a turtle we mistook for a land mine on the road. Hard times and horror had been part of these women's daily lives. It showed in their eyes and in their hesitant manners. They each carried scars, cauterized deep in body memory.

"Come on. Come on. Help me out. What did I say?" I begged. I didn't really care if they were laughing at me. It was so good just to hear them laugh.

Hamide was just beginning to study the English language. Sometimes in the evening she stayed after the others left, and we practiced simple conversations. Only the night before she taught me a touching sentence: *Kam shprese*. It means, "I have hope." Now she enjoyed teasing her teacher.

"Miss Nancy, how many peaches . . . you do have?" Hamide asked.

"Good sentence, Hamide!" I replied. I counted the fruit on the tray. "It looks like I have five."

This set the group into hysterics. They laughed so hard they could barely talk. Nurse Dijetare translated what I had said for Dr. Drita, who then laughed so hard she nearly wet herself as she ran for the bathroom.

"Are you guys going to tell me what it means?" I asked again just as Dr. Drita returned from the bathroom. Drita said something in Albanian to Bedrije. She seemed to be saying they should include the American in the joke.

"No! Not me! Dijetare, tell her," Bedrije said, laughing as she passed the buck to her friend.

"No! Hamide, you tell her," Dijetare replied, covering her face with her hands.

"No! Not me! Dr, Mirvete," Hamide shrieked, cheeks braising red.

Dr. Mirvete just shook her head and continued to howl.

Finally, blushing through her laughter as she wiped her tears away, Bedrije said, "Miss Nancy, in our country we call the word *peaches*. . ." Then she covered her face with one hand and pointed to her crotch with the other, sending the group into another spasm of laughter.

It was a good joke on me. I laughed along with the other women until finally, gasping for breath, I managed to say, "Oh, I guess then I only have one," which sent everyone into another laughing fit.

I was awed by the strength of these women. They each had lived through their own private hell, before and during the war, but now they persistently worked to rebuild their lives and their country. And the fact that they could howl with laughter together on this hot afternoon gave me hope that maybe—just maybe—both they and their country could begin to heal. I heard Hamide's voice in my head whisper. . . *Hope is life. Life is hope. Kam shprese*. I have hope.

My Little Lamp

~

Bonnie Jarvis-Lowe, RN

Newspapers cluttered the floors, the furniture was topsy-turvy, cardboard boxes were stashed everywhere: our house was in a state of complete chaos. It was moving time again. We were packing our things and relocating to a place we both loved so much, Newfoundland.

We had lived in Nova Scotia all our married lives—33 years and a few months—more time than we had lived in Newfoundland. It's a beautiful province, with a wonderful people and great climate, and we had made many friends over the years.

But it was time to come home. Never had we planned it, never discussed it at any length.

Through all of the years in various towns in Nova Scotia, we worked, contributed to the community, and had good lives. But now the treadmill was a little too fast and we seemed to be on a fast train to nowhere. We had too much house and too much work. We watched friends in their late forties and early fifties die, and I had to make a change or I felt I would wither and die without ever getting in a boat, going out on the bay, catching a fish, or having the experience of living near my sisters.

So we made plans to retire. My nursing career was so precious to me, though, that the decision was very difficult. My husband led the way and taught me to move on, not to look back with regret.

We placed our house on the market, thinking that in a few months or so it would sell. It was June, so we would have the summer to make all sorts of preparations. That was not to be, because the house sold the same day it was listed.

So the rush was on to get moving—and quickly. The farewells, the summer's heat, running out of time, selling off things that had become just burdensome . . . it was all very physically taxing and bittersweet.

One day, in the middle of all the upheaval, even though pushed for time, I took a precious possession off the shelf and sat on the crowded sofa with it in my hands. The tears rolled down my face as I carefully held and brushed the dust off the dear old lamp.

It was a kerosene oil lamp that had been mine for many years. It was in a metal stand, or hanger, with a hole in the back for hanging on a wall. It stood 16 inches high, with a fragile glass chimney that was 14 inches around the widest part. A decorative pattern in white ran around that widest part of the chimney and a shiny reflector was mounted on the metal holder. When lit, the light would reflect beautifully, doubling the effect of the flame.

This was no ordinary lamp.

WHEN I WAS a student at the Grace General Hospital School of Nursing from 1966 to 1969, I, of course, had to do a stint in the well-baby nursery as part of obstetrics, and I loved it. I was 18 years old in 1967, and Mrs. Smallwood was the head nurse in the nursery on the second floor. One day she was going through a closet and all these lamps were sitting in a row on a shelf. I asked her about them.

She told me stories of being a student herself, of those lamps hanging on the walls, of nurses feeding the babies in the middle of the night by the lamplight, and of the beautiful picture it brought to her mind. I picked a lamp off the shelf and asked her what they would do with them now.

"Oh, I suppose they'll go to the dump. Nobody cares about them now," she replied.

"Well, I do," I remarked.

"Well, Jarvis, if you want one, take it. It's yours! But promise to take care of it!"

I promised I would do just that and walked away with my little lamp.

Little did I know that my lamp would follow me to Grand Bank, St. John's, and various places in Nova Scotia, and would always occupy a special spot in my home wherever I was. Many people would ask about it, many people admired it, and the most amazing thing of all is that through all the moves, all the packing and tossing around, it never, ever broke!

IT SITS HERE on my desk as I write today, back in Newfoundland: My lamp and I, still together.

It was used once or twice during power failures when winter storms hit. It was knocked off a shelf by someone looking behind it for a book. It was in a box that a moving van lost, but was eventually found and returned to me still unbroken.

So I sat in my chaotic household that day and held my lamp. To me it signified my life, my career, and my own resilience that at times I thought was gone. I carefully—very carefully—packed it for the journey back to Newfoundland.

Maybe some cold winter evening, I will trim the wick again and light my lamp. And maybe I'll see the image of nurses in starchy white uniforms feeding the babies under that golden glow. The lamp has lasted and stood the test of time, and now it's up to me to see if I too can stand the test of time.

A Lesson in the Elusiveness of Hope

~

Laura Monahan

IN ONE OF my first weeks in clinical rounds as a new student nurse, I was assigned to a patient, JS, who had diabetes (with its many complications) and advanced stage multiple myeloma. JS had chemotherapy two years ago and had recently been transferred from another hospital because of compression on the cervical vertebrae 4, 5, and 6. He had a Hartmann's procedure colonoscopy that was still healing and a large sacral ulcer that was not progressing well. He had been at the hospital for more than a month, and on the day that I was taking care of him, a team of cancer doctors arrived to meet with him and his wife to discuss his options.

The oncology doctors told JS that there was really nothing more they could do for him. Additional chemotherapy wouldn't be productive, and their objective at this point in time was just to make him as comfortable as possible to the end. I happened to be in the room with JS when the doctors arrived, and it was almost surreal listening to them. It was as if time had stopped, frozen, and each second stood as an eternity unto itself. The words seemed to hang starkly and forebodingly in midair; they sliced hope into ribbons of a past, unattainable reality, with a foreign and alternate eternity superimposed upon the present one.

The doctors told JS, in essence, that this was the end of the road. All that was left for him was to face death as the ultimate option; did he understand that? The only thing they could do now was help him manage his pain. JS cried. His wife cried. I wanted to cry and scream and rage, to be anywhere else than that hospital room at that moment.

Each week after clinical, our assignment was to write up a clinical data sheet on our patient and his or her health status for that week. I had a hard time processing what I had experienced that week. As I wrote the clinical data sheet on JS that weekend, I couldn't stop weeping. Every time I sat down to write, my eyes filled with tears, and I felt such an overwhelming sense of loss, helplessness, and frustration. It was a crushing burden of sadness.

My husband was baffled. This was not like me. He kept asking me what was wrong. I had hardly even known this patient, why I was so upset? Who was this man, really, to me? My husband questioned whether nursing was the right career for me. Perhaps I had made a mistake in not going to law school instead? I had been accepted into several impressive law schools. Had I made a mistake in not pursuing that avenue instead?

I didn't know what to tell him and began to wonder too if I had made a grievous mistake. Every time I thought about JS, I felt so powerless, so ineffective. There was nothing I could do to fix the situation. I had come from a business and management background, and I was used to fixing things. That was my modus operandi: if something wasn't right, I worked like the devil until it was.

Nursing, I found, though, was not like business. In business if you worked really, really hard, you accomplished your goals and even turned the tide if things were going badly. The losses too were so much less: even if you had lost millions of dollars, there was still life, still breath; there was still the opportunity to recoup losses on another more favorable day.

But the loss of life, its breath, and all its scope of opportunities—that was much more permanent, static, and nonnegotiable. It was a hard, concrete reality there was no way of outmaneuvering. How could you barter with death? You couldn't negotiate best options, no matter how much drive, creativity, and resources you had at your disposal. There was no way you could work out a best-alternatives scenario to negotiated agreement with your adversary. Death was a cold and implacable opponent, and I, in the end, was facing this. It was a brick wall. All the tools at my disposal, all the talents I had previously used with such success and bravado, came to naught here. There was nothing I could do in this situation, except face it and accept it as a nonnegotiable reality. Sadly, I didn't know what else to do.

At church on Sunday, in desperation, I prayed for JS, pleading with God to take him into his care, to alleviate his pain and sorrow. I asked my husband, Jim, and daughter, Gaby, to say extra prayers for JS and his family during this time of their sorrow. Although I felt their loss, I had a hard time processing it. I began to question whether I had the courage to face this new world of nursing that I had somehow stumbled blindly into.

My clinical instructor, Julie, sat down with me the following week and helped me address my fears. She said that, although there are many difficult moments in nursing, as a nurse you were an advocate for your patient and a valuable resource for facing those difficult—and often desperate—moments. Nurses could not always take the pain completely away, but we could ease the burden of that pain and help patients, as compassionate companions, along in their journey. Nurses were often guides along those tempestuous and precarious ways, like sea captains navigating restless seas. Nurses greeted people as they came into the world and bade them off with courage as they left. There was no other profession with such honor, she said, and although it took stamina and conviction, it was well worth the effort through the lives you touched, enriched, and yes, even saved.

Her words gave me courage to not give up and press on, to fight the good fight without looking back. Even though at this point in time I only know enough to keep putting one foot in front of the other, my hope is to fulfill this role with the grace, courage, and tenacity that I see in other nurses, however elusive the happy ending.

Poetry as Hope

~

Mary H. Palmer, PhD, RNC, FAAN

As a nurse and part of a family with several members living with chronic illness, I have often turned to literature—especially poetry—that gives voice to the suffering, longing for healing, and hope. It acts as a balm and it acts as a source for insight and empathy. One poet, Jane Kenyon, used writing as a means to make visible the suffering and hope of people living with serious chronic illnesses.

Kenyon suffered from depressive episodes that permeated her life. She was not diagnosed with bipolar disease until she was 38 years old, although she was aware of her depression from childhood. She described living with depression as, "You're like a chipmunk on the eagle's talons." Despite her illness, the creative force to examine, to explore, and to express never left her. She said in an interview, "For me poetry's a safe place always, a refuge." She went on to say that she believed a poet is a namer of names, but that a poet must bring consolation, even by doing nothing more than putting emotions into words.

Many of Kenyon's poems focus on nature, and they are suffused with images and metaphors that describe her illness. They also describe the redemption and relief from spiritual pain that comes through love, beauty, hope, and prayer. In "Peonies at Dusk," she writes, "In the darkening June evening / I draw a blossom near, and bending close / search it as a woman searches / a loved one's face." Perhaps this is why her poetry resonates with me: the garden acts as a place of refuge and realization I return to time and again. The awareness that the fulsome and colorful blossoms of early summer ultimately yield to short gray days of winter only makes these blossoms all the more precious. The life cycle is inescapable in a garden: next to full flowers are those starting to droop as they shed petals and seeds. By stopping, searching, and taking stock, I am allowed to see the detail in the expansiveness. Stepping out of my situation, grace flows in and that grace will lead to action. Hope allows me to find the boat that will take me back to shore. It helps me help others.

Another of my favorite Kenyon poems, "Biscuit," examines the relationship between the powerful and powerless, the roles of hope and faith, and the responsibility the powerful have toward the powerless, by invoking one of the most sacred points of Catholic Mass, Communion. Told in first person, the simple story of feeding a dog a biscuit as a reward for finishing its meal is transformed into a powerful story. It unfolds as a story of unquestioning faith ("He asks for bread, expects / bread . . .").

The tenderness of the speaker's voice resonates throughout the poem. It is easy to identify with the speaker when she says, " . . . and I in my power / might have given him a stone," while looking into the upturned face and luminous dark eyes of a dog expecting a treat. Everyone has experienced that split second, that instant before responding to an entrusting request. We can give an endearing response or we can spurn the request and do injury. It is in this coming together—the requester's faith and the goodness of the person to whom the request is made—that communion occurs.

"Biscuit" is also a condensed statement about the sacredness of the bond between two creatures and their interdependence. This poem contrasts the views of the ill speaker who knows that the future is full of pitfalls, perhaps even more suffering, and the healthy dog that is oblivious to any barriers to achieving his reward. Kenyon's speaker says in this poem, "I can't bear that trusting face!"

Kenyon is also saying that when one trusts, vulnerability exists. Mutual awareness and acceptance of this vulnerability is a painful and sacred trust. Nurses often work with awareness and acceptance of this vulnerability. We enter the intimate world of a suffering other and make attempts to bring hope by relieving or alleviating that suffering. We are aware that people turn to us as a source of hope, and we in turn draw strength from the hope that emanates from them.

Throughout her poems Kenyon employs powerful metaphors to describe potent and destructive diseases and the personal struggle against those diseases. She extracts elements from everyday life, holds them under the microscope of the poetic eye, and then she offers the results for all to inspect. In this process, she illustrates the obvious and simple, creates something new, and exposes the hidden complexities of the human heart and its response to the world.

By reading Kenyon's poems as well as writings by other authors who explore the human condition, nurses have the opportunity to pause and see what is visible. And in doing so, we see both the struggle to find communion that can come with illness and the enduring nature of hope.

Alice

~

Patricia Harman, RN, CNM, MSN

"Fine . . . fine," Alice says. "Been just fine," she replies to my questioning. She is here for her yearly gyn exam and speaks with a mountain twang. "Ain't got time to be sick!" I study the woman, appreciating her. Alice Corkney is a tough old bird, in her seventies, the kind of woman who's had a hard life and it shows. Some of her teeth are missing, the ones on the side that show when she grins.

I go through my list of questions. "Any vaginal bleeding?"

"Not for some time!" the patient chuckles.

"Bowel or bladder problems? Any new health problems in you or the family?" I ask.

"No. No. No. Doing just fine."

I get down to the sex question, think of skipping it, but don't. "So are you married, Alice?" This is my lead-in.

"Sure am, 40 years this spring. He's a good man too. Used to work in the mines until his health broke."

"Are you still sexually active?"

"No, not hardly, honey. It's the man, you know. He's disabled. I pretty much have to take care of him now."

"I guess I didn't know that. What's his trouble?"

"He can't get around much. He has that muscular dystrophy. If we have to go somewhere he uses a walker, but I pretty much have to wait on him." She looks like she doesn't mind, looks almost proud. "Him and my son too."

"Your son *too*? What's wrong with *him*?"

"Same thing. The muscle thing. It's the inherited kind. There's medicine, but we can't get it. Too expensive. We tried to get a state medical card, but it was so much running into town for interviews, we just gave up. Because we own the farm, we probably wouldn't qualify anyway."

"So your son stays home with you? How old is he?"

"Yeah, he still lives with me and Pap. We're used to it. He's 31." It's a slow day in the clinic so I take my time. How the woman thinks interests me; what her life is like.

I start her exam at the top and work my way to her bottom. Alice's breasts hang on her front. They'd been full once. The cut of her muscles shows under her loose, wrinkled skin. We talk as I continue. "Looks like you do some farmwork."

Alice laughs. It's more of a cackle. "We still keep a cow. Love that fresh milk. But the work's mostly mine now. I pretty much run the farm."

"Can't Bobbie help you?"

"Oh, he does the milking, but I do the other stuff. You know. Feeding. Cleaning the stalls in the winter when it's too bad to let the cow out. I have to do the heavy lifting. His legs ain't that strong." She has a cheery way of saying all this.

"So, does it ever get you down? It seems like you're carrying the whole family."

"No, I'm fine. It's what God gave me," she says simply.

Alice doesn't complain, but I complain all the time, complain about the patients when they are late, complain about shrinking reimbursement from insurance companies, complain about the rising cost of malpractice insurance.

When the snow comes in sideways, wet and hard, coating the trunks of trees, Alice stomps her way to the barn and milks the one cow. All over the earth, good people toil like this, happy to be alive and carry their load.

I would bow down to Alice, but she'd only laugh.

A Silent Woman

~

Eileen Valinoti, RN

THE PATIENT, A middle-aged woman, lay huddled in bed in a fetal position, lost in a catatonic stupor. The side rails were locked in place. Someone had put the call light in the woman's hand, where it rested against her inert palm.

"Jane," the head nurse said, bending down close to the patient and speaking into her ear as if she were deaf, "here is your nurse, *Miss Kelly*." The nurse was smiling and she said my name so liltingly, in a tone of such buoyant hope, that one would think I had come to offer a cure.

The patient only stared at us, her eyes blank and unseeing. She gave no sign that she had heard, not a flicker of an eyelash nor a quiver of her lips. Only the soft sounds of her regular breathing indicated life.

"They're waiting for a bed on psychiatry," the head nurse whispered to me, explaining why Jane was on our busy medical surgical unit.

"She may be here for a couple of days," she said over her shoulder as she hurried out the door and disappeared down the hall.

I was 20 years old, a senior nursing student, with little knowledge of psychiatry. I hardly knew what catatonia was. At the nurses' station, I read Jane's chart, hoping for some guidance. There was a brief history: the patient had been found motionless on her couch at home by a concerned neighbor who hadn't seen her in days. At first the neighbor thought she was dead. An ambulance had taken the patient to the emergency room where she was seen by the psychiatric resident. *Severe depression*, he had written. That was all. I saw at once that I would have to learn on the job, as it were. In those days, over 40 years ago, nursing education was really an apprenticeship with patients themselves our unwitting teachers and mentors.

When I went back into Jane's room, she lay in the same frozen posture. I had a sinking feeling of inadequacy, of apprehension. What approach did one take with this patient? I had no idea.

I took refuge in the familiar rituals of bedside care, bathing her and putting clean sheets on the bed, then changing her gown. I had to struggle to ease her stiff limbs into the armholes; her muscles were so stiff and unyielding. She felt as lifeless as a mannequin. I thought of the large doll we had practiced on in our nursing arts classroom—Mrs. Chase, we called her. Jane had the same vacant, impenetrable gaze, the same aura of profound indifference.

The patient had long, thick dark hair that spilled out all over the pillow. I brushed and combed it, trying to disentangle the knots, wanting her to look neat, presentable in case her teenage son visited. He had come once when she was admitted; I had seen him standing far away from the bed, looking at her with horrified eyes and clenching and unclenching his fists.

I tried to move Jane's woodenlike legs in the circular motion we called "bicycle exercises." I was afraid of blood clots forming in the large vessels in her calves. Would she notice a feeling of heat, a throbbing or even pain? I didn't know, but she wouldn't complain if she did.

When I finished, I made futile attempts to feed the patient.

"Jane," I said, my voice loud as if to arouse her, "it's time to eat." Holding the spoon in my hand while the untouched food grew sodden, I felt hopeless, helpless. I worried about the other patients I was assigned to care for—who were waiting for me now, restless in damp, rumpled beds, needing to be refreshed, gotten up, walked. It was a busy unit and I was always falling behind. In the hallway, nurses rushed by with trays of syringes, doctors hurried past, their long white coats flapping behind them, clergymen bearing breviaries stepped smartly, but here in this room all was hushed and still.

I was assigned to Jane every day. She never gave me the slightest sign of recognition, remaining as affectless as the furniture in the room, her face as blank as the unadorned white walls. I spoke to her anyway, knowing she wouldn't answer.

"That's better," I would murmur while washing her face or, "You'll be warmer now," when I pulled the blanket over her shoulders, talking to her as one does to a very young child or to an infant, in the vague hope that my voice might reach the subterranean depths where the patient lived. I pulled the shades up high, letting in the light. The sunshine would be good for her, I thought. She was so pale, her face as white as the bedsheets. An IV dripped steadily into her arm, keeping her firmly tethered to this world.

Few people came into the room. The cleaning woman would mop the floor quickly, casting anxious glances at the woman in the bed. The psychiatric resident appeared briefly to put his stethoscope to Jane's thin chest and listen intently, his head cocked to one side. The head nurse stopped in to inquire about Jane's blood pressure.

"You're checking the vital signs?" she asked me.

"Yes," I would say, showing her the sheet where I recorded everything: temperature, pulse, and blood pressure, all written in neat columns, proving that Jane was alive.

Her teenage son did not return. I couldn't blame him. There was a feeling of such anguishing sadness in the room that your heart rose up in your throat. In the other patients' rooms, laughter could rise up even out of abject misery. A cancer-ridden patient, an emaciated blonde who chain-smoked and talked constantly, joked with us about finding the night nurse asleep at the desk—"Her snoring woke me up," she told us. A 90-year-old Irish nun loved to tell us the story of her rescue as a child from the sinking *Lusitania*. In the icy ocean, clinging to the wreckage, she promised God she would join the convent if she were saved. When we had her swallow the pills she hated, she would turn up her nose and say in her high-pitched voice, "You tinkers," an Irish term of opprobrium and scorn.

IT WAS EARLY spring and when I looked out the windows of Jane's room, I could see a few stalwart trees on the bleak city street spouting soft green leaves. I was looking forward to my weekend off when my boyfriend and I would ride our bikes in Central Park. In the airless room, I imagined how good the cool wind would feel in my face as we rode together beneath the trees.

When I had finished taking care of Jane, she looked clean and tidy, her dry lips moistened with lemon and glycerin, her hair brushed back from her face, her IV neatly in place. In those days, we set great store by appearances. Neatness counted, never mind death and despair. I told Jane I was leaving for a while, but that I would be back. She never raised an eyebrow or arched her neck even slightly as I rushed out the door, anxious to complete my work.

On Monday, when I returned from my days off, people were rushing about more than usual. There was a flu going around and two nurses had called in sick. We had no replacements; everyone would have to double up.

"Jane's going to the psych unit today," the head nurse whispered to me. Then she added, "We've got two new admissions; both stab wounds from a fight in one of the neighborhood bars. It'll be a madhouse here today."

That was fine with me. I felt strong, energetic, and rejuvenated by the afternoons in Central Park with my boyfriend, among the other cheerful bicyclists and chattering families. We had ridden on the merry-go-round alongside laughing children, eaten frankfurters at the hot dog stand, made faces at the monkeys in the zoo.

I went to the linen closet to get my supplies. In my head, I was counting the days until I saw my boyfriend again. Then, as I walked from the closet into the hallway, I saw Jane. She was advancing down the hall, gaunt and dazed, leaning heavily on the arm of the nurse's aide, a sturdy-looking Hispanic woman. It seemed that she was being propelled rather than walking freely. She had on a navy blue bathrobe and slippers, and she was wearing large horn-rimmed eyeglasses. She looked like any ordinary middle-aged woman except for the startled look she had, as if she had been suddenly jolted awake. With great care and concentration, she put one foot in front of the other, keeping pace with the nurse's aide. Her demeanor was that of a person who is eager to please, to cooperate, to do what is expected, while at the same time trying to puzzle out what that might be. A doctor on his rounds turned and stared curiously.

As I stood in the hall watching, Jane suddenly broke away from the nurse's aide and walked toward me, taking stiff, jerky steps and staring fixedly ahead like a sleepwalker. She reached out and touched my arm.

"Thank you," she said. Her voice was hoarse and the words came out in an effortful monotone, as if she were struggling to remember the phrase in a foreign language. Her hand felt cold through the thin cotton of my uniform sleeve. I was so startled, so stunned, that I recoiled, stepping backwards and almost losing my balance. Some of the sheets and pillowcases in my arms fell to the floor. I started to say something, but then the aide took Jane's arm, the elevator came, and they got on it together, merging into the small crowd of patients and visitors.

Spontaneous Acts of
Kindness

~

K. Lynn Wieck, PhD, RN

A FEW YEARS AGO, a letter arrived at our home. It wasn't even addressed to me; it was for our son who was away at college. The return address was a home just down the street. Thinking our son had backed over someone's begonias again, I opened the letter to find out the damage.

The letter turned out to be a solicitation. One of my neighbors was chairing the Leukemia Society drive in our neighborhood and wanted to know if we would donate. I was so relieved her begonias were still intact that I decided to write a check right then and there.

I slapped the modest check into the return envelope she had included, attached a stamp that she had not included, and then paused for a moment.

I thought about how much we in health care depend on people just like my neighbor to raise the funds to sponsor research for the elimination of diseases. I also thought about how busy I think I am and how glad I was that I was not in charge of getting donations. So I grabbed a handy sticky note and a pen and wrote this small note:

Mrs. X,

I want to thank you for taking your time and energy to raise money in our neighborhood to fight leukemia. I am a nurse, and we get to see the good that the money you raise does in helping little kids who would have died just a few short generations ago. I know you have a lot of other things you could do, so I just want to tell you how much I appreciate you. Enclosed is my check to help this cause.

In admiration,
Lynn Wieck.

The whole thing took less than a minute or two. I stuck the note to the check and sent the letter on its way. I didn't even take the check to her; I let the mail carrier do the legwork. I never gave it another thought.

A few weeks later, I received a call in the early evening hours. The voice asked to speak to me. I immediately went into my "anti-phone-solicitor" mode, but she informed me she was my neighbor. Figuring *I* had creamed someone's flowers this time, I switched to my "sorry—it was an accident" mode.

Here's what she said: "I just moved to this community a few months ago. I am retired and have been doing solicitation drives for several charities for over 18 years. I just want you to know how much I appreciate your note. In 18 years, this is the first time anyone ever thanked me for asking them for money."

We had a nice chat—short, friendly, uplifting. When she hung up, I knew she felt good. The endorphins were raging. There was happiness in the air. And I thought about how this spontaneous little act had triggered something so good.

What do you think Mrs. X believes about nurses based on this incident? I hope she thinks they are nice, kind, polite, mannerly, and grateful. When Mrs. X's extremely bright and gifted granddaughter comes for Christmas this year and says, "You know Grandma, I think I want to be a nurse," what do you think she'll say as she gazes at this darling child who is the light of her grandparents' eyes? Maybe she'll say, "Yes, dear, that sounds perfect for you."

Who knows? My point is that people remember things. They remember the nurse who was rude to them in the emergency room, the nurse who made them leave the ICU when Grandpa was so sick, the nurse who was too busy to pull the sheets tight so Johnny could sleep. So why wouldn't they remember the nice things too?

I share this story because I know that thousands of you perform this exact same type of spontaneous kindness every day. You probably think no one is watching and that no one cares. I beg to differ. Someone is always watching, and everyone cares. We have such a wonderful opportunity to sell our profession when we engage in spontaneous acts of kindness as nurses. Nursing attracts kind and generous people who care about others.

Life is in overdrive today. The pace is fast, and if you slow down, you might get run over. This chaos and frenzy is making us tired. It is also crowding out the little things we do that make such a big difference.

My biggest fear is that we will lose the energy and will to perform these spontaneous acts of kindness that make the public (as well as ourselves) feel good about nursing and about life itself. It would be terrible to cheat ourselves out of the pleasure that comes with being kind to others, even when no one is looking.

I want to be presumptuous enough to thank each of you for your spontaneous acts of kindness on behalf of all nurses. You make us look good. You make nursing an attractive career alternative. And you contribute to your own sense of self-worth. Those huge benefits are worth a few minutes of our time any day.

Intersection

~

Elizabeth Tibbetts, RN

WHEN I WAS a young maternity nurse still fresh with all I had learned in school, I walked into a patient's room and told her a truth about myself. I'd been taught not to do this: not to cross the line between professional and personal. I'd taken this advice seriously and approached my patients with full attention to their lives and needs. I was careful to leave the details of my own life at home. I happily attended women and their families through labor and birth, taught them to feed and care for their babies, listened to their worries. In the intimacy of that setting, many patients asked about me. I would say I had a son, or talk about my garden and the town I lived in. But I would never say much about my hectic life as a single mother trying to work and take care of my child.

Then a high school girl came in, the daughter of a professional couple in the community. Her doctor told the nurses she would be giving her baby up for adoption. He told us she did not want to hold the baby after birth, and no one was to visit except her family. The girl gave birth to a boy, and then stayed in her room with the door closed. The baby stayed in the nursery, swaddled and rocked by us nurses until he could go with his adoptive family. I wrapped his mother's breasts, iced her stitches, tended everything I could for her, and then listened.

She told a story of falling for a local boy and then finding herself pregnant. She said her parents wanted her to give the baby up and she had agreed it would be best; she could then head off to college and the rest of her life. She had agreed it would be too hard to see her baby and that the father would not see the baby, either. She said this was the right decision. As she spoke, her voice was quiet and matter-of-fact, the expression in her eyes remote.

Her parents visited. They were attentive and clearly loved their daughter. And they reinforced that she had made the right decision. We were reminded of all the restrictions. When the baby's father and his family tried to visit, as we had been warned they would, we turned them away. And although we nurses thought the girl might feel better if she saw her baby, had a chance to meet him and say good-bye, we did not say this to her. The baby stayed in the nursery for two days. On the third day the girl asked to hold him, to see him once. She crooked the baby in her arms, smiled, and started to cry as she looked at his fingers, then his toes, and into his wide eyes. Then she sent the baby back. Later in the day she asked to hold him again. When her parents visited we explained that this was her right. They talked with her. She agreed that the adoption would proceed.

The next day she held the baby again. I poked my head into her room to check on them. She was cradling him against her chest, and there was such a look on her face: the expression of someone who has seen a situation they cannot bear. She looked up at me and said, "I told my parents I would give him up. I know it makes the most sense." And then she added, "But he's so beautiful—I don't know what to do anymore." The nurse I was taught to be listened. I was quiet as she talked and cried. And then the person I was—beyond being a nurse—stepped further into the room, opened my mouth and said, "I was in a similar situation once." That's all. As soon as the words popped out of my mouth, I was afraid that I had overstepped. The words were out. I couldn't retract them. But the girl looked right at me, and something changed. A spark that I hadn't seen before flickered in her eyes—as though she had seen possibility or hope or her way through a difficult situation. In an urgent voice she asked me a series of yes or no questions. It was as though she sensed I could not elaborate, so she quickly asked what she had to know. Had I kept the baby? Was I still married? Was I glad I'd kept my baby?

That afternoon she called the baby's father. He arrived in his carpenter's clothes and was careful to wash his hands. He and the girl sat in the bed together laughing and crying as they admired their son. They talked fast, making plans, plans the girl would have to explain to her worried parents. They were so young. Their lives would not be easy. That girl would have to work hard to reach any semblance of the life she had imagined before all of this had happened. But she had the straight-on look of a girl who had looked clearly at her choices and made one.

I never heard what happened after they left the hospital. But I still wonder about that girl now that my own son is grown and has children of his own. Though I didn't tell her more, the similarities between her circumstance and my own were uncanny, so close that I could not stop myself from speaking, could not stand the hollow look in her eyes of someone who does not believe in what they're about to do. At the time

I wasn't sure I should have spoken those few words, words that may have changed the course of my patient's life. But I had done what felt right: letting her know, in the most personal way, that she had a choice.

And after nearly 30 years of nursing, I have come to believe that healing takes place in the tender, personal intersection between people. That those moments, when we share our humanness, may be the moments when people find peace, healing, understanding, or clarity. And I truly hope wherever that girl—now woman—is, that she is well and thriving.

The Rules

~

Barbara Gordon Sauvage, RN

You get points for visiting people in the hospital. Well, you get points for visiting sick people, anyway. You're not supposed to feel good about getting points; they take points away if you feel good about getting them. Okay, you're not supposed to feel good about being good, either, even if you were good for the hell of it and not because you wanted the points. You're never supposed to feel good. Good is bad. Got that? Welcome to Catholic Childhood Hell.

So when you do something good, you feel bad, because you did something good and you're not supposed to feel good about it. Then you feel bad about doing something good, and the next time you want to do something good, you think twice about it, because why, after all, do you *want* to do something good if it's bad to feel good?

So you get to be, oh, say, 47 ½ years old, and you wonder: why do I give a rat's ass about feeling good or feeling bad, and why am I always second-guessing my motives based on crap I learned in the first grade? Why, oh why?

So you go back to basics: reeducate yourself, like that's even remotely possible, but even after all the good-bad-good-bad stuff, you have to sit yourself down and say, okay, I'm a grown-up now. I can do good stuff and feel bad about it. I can do bad stuff and feel good about it. Just figure out what you're supposed to be doing with yourself, with your life, with the people you love, and thank God you're still able to *do that* even if *God* was the reason you felt so goddamn bad in the first place. But oh well, it's a crazy universe we live in with crazy rules. And hey—I didn't make the rules; I just play by them.

Or I don't.

So you visit your friend in the hospital, and she is dying and crazy because the cancer is in her brain now. You visit this friend with your other friend who is an evangelical born-again Christian, who also feels bad about being good because we're all basically bad anyway. You force yourself to visit nonetheless because, goddamnit, it's the *right* thing and the *good* thing to do. Got that?

So you visit Clive, who is as good as they get, but not namby-pamby about it because after all, she is a 65-year-old black woman from Mississippi who was orphaned at four and M'Deara raised her to believe you *just do it* and be done with it—good, bad, or indifferent.

Clive says to me one night—when we worked nights on hospice together—that she was married at 16 and that lasted four years, and she was married again in her twenties to some guy that cheated on her and she dumped him, and then she met William, with whom she has been shacking up on or off for some 20-odd years and "Shacking, Barb, is just fine."

For the last five years, though, she and William have been legal. I think they just wanted to straighten out the financial situation finally, and William is sitting over in the chair and we're talking about Ramsey Lewis, who is working with the music students at Roosevelt, where my daughter is going to school.

"You know, Roosevelt," Clive says to William.

"Franklin Roosevelt?" I say.

"No, another Roosevelt," says Clive.

I tell them about my baby playing the "Star Spangled Banner" at graduation, old-school jazz style, and "Lover Man" at the high school concert. I hum a few bars and William remembers the tune, and Clive is sitting in a Geri chair and I am giving her a foot rub.

WHEN I WALKED into the hospital room and saw Clive, she was not making a lot of sense, and I was real, real sad about that, because even when Clive didn't make sense in the past, she still made more sense than most of the people I know on a good day—including me. She said that she didn't know Gail or me, but I could see in her eyes that she did—or at least that at some point it would dawn on her during the visit. I sat next to Clive and Gail sat next to me. Clive said she was seeing white fleas and asked William if he saw them too. He said no, and Gail said, "It's the pressure on her brain," and I said, "The tumor is pressing on her eyes," and then thought, enough of the shoptalk. Clive tried to say something about not making sense—and she wasn't—and I said, "It's the disease, don't worry about it." But of course, we all worried about it, even though worrying about it at this stage of the game is a day late and a dollar short, but oh well, that's what we humans do up 'til the end. I thought, time for plan B, so I sidled up close to Clive and said, "Hey, how do you like this shirt?"

And she glanced at my sleeve and said in a low voice, "I love that shirt."

"I stole it from my husband," I said. "Hey, that shirt doesn't look good on you. Let me try it on."

Gail said she liked William's shirt, and I said I'd steal that too after he went to sleep.

I asked Clive if she remembered my bad foot and the hammertoe. She had told me to get me some big old shoes, that my shoes were too tight, and she took me shopping to "the big folks' shoe place." I stuck my foot up on the tray attached to the Geri chair that stopped Clive from trying to get up and just falling down again, and showed her my surgical shoe with my toe sticking up with the fake pearl on top of the pin stuck in the toe to keep it straight while it healed—a perfectly understandable gesture to someone with brain mets.

I said to her, "Do you want me to give you a foot massage?" Clive, who never wants anyone to do anything for her, said, "Not necessarily. You can if you want to."

So I switched places with Gail, and William rifled through the drawer and came up with some lotion, and I started rubbing Clive's feet—felt good about rubbing Clive's feet. I mean, Jesus did that at the Last Supper, and then I felt bad about rubbing Clive's feet because I felt good about it. But I continued to do it because, damn it all, it was the right thing to do. I looked out into the hall and the tall deacon, the grief minister resembling Ichabod Crane, walked by and I smiled at him. He doesn't remember me, I thought, can't place me; I worked with him for four years. None of us can place each other anymore; only Clive truly remembers us somewhere in the back of her head where the cancer doesn't live.

Gail held Clive's hand. Clive grabbed the lotion and told Gail her hands needed a little work, so I rubbed Clive's feet while Clive rubbed Gail's hands, because Clive doesn't believe in getting something for nothing. I looked at William and said, "One night when we were working together, we walked into this patient's room. He had had surgery for pancreatic cancer and a 12-inch suture line that had opened up. You could see into his abdomen."

William said, "Couldn't they sew it up again?"

"Nope," I said, "wouldn't hold. Sometimes it doesn't."

Anyway, this guy had this jury-rigged clear garbage bag thing that was about four feet long and emptied into a pail taped to his abdomen. When he drank a glass of water, the water poured out of the hole in his stomach down through the plastic shoot and into the pail. I was truly amazed; that was one of the most screwed-up things I'd ever seen up until then. It was like looking into the invisible-man toy in Don's dime store when I was a kid, the one with the see-through skin and all the organs visible. You could take them out and reassemble them again. God, I wanted that toy! You've got to belong to the Addams Family to be a really good nurse. Anyhow, the adhesive on his skin had come loose, and Clive sat there and cut up more DuoDERM to patch around the opening and talked to this guy like nothing was wrong, just sat there like she was making a dress. "Were you a big drinker?" she asked him. "Yeah," he said.

I told William, "She's a good nurse."

William said, "She always liked going to work. But she didn't like getting up in the morning."

I asked Clive if she wanted me to bring her something special to eat the next time I came.

"She don't eat much," William said.

"Only a few bites then I'm done," Clive said. "But don't worry—if you want to bring something go ahead and bring it."

DON'T FEEL BAD about it, that's all. That's one of the rules.

Mr. Bunyan

~

Madeleine Mysko, RN

AFTER HIS WIFE died, he sold their home and moved into an apartment in our independent living wing. Already he was in trouble: congestive heart failure, edema, shortness of breath, and nasty skin eruptions in places he couldn't reach when he bathed, which wasn't often. Moreover, there were unexplained scrapes and bruises—evidence he'd suffered a couple of falls, though he vehemently denied it. He should have been packed up and moved to the health care center weeks earlier, where he would have received the nursing care he needed. But he wasn't the sort of man anyone just packed up and moved.

He was in trouble, and we both knew it, but only one of us was going to admit it. That would have been me: the "new" nurse recently graduated from the RN refresher course, the one cheerfully determined to deliver the very best practice in geriatric nursing, the one he consistently addressed as "lady," as in "Ask you something, lady—do your people ever communicate with each other?" or "Listen, lady—nobody's going to pull the wool over these eyes."

He was a big man. I'll call him Paul Bunyan, because sometimes when I visited him—when he was still able to draw himself to full height—he'd tower over me like the fabled lumberjack. Also, he had a favorite flannel shirt that he wore year-round—red, a lumberjack plaid.

Once upon a time, Mr. Bunyan applied his engineering acumen and his big, capable hands to overseeing the maintenance of an entire complex of university buildings. But age and sickness put an end to that. And so he wasn't as good-humored as the storybook character. Sometimes he could be really mean. I would walk the eighth-floor hall toward his door, brace myself, and pause to take a breath before lifting the knocker. Though he'd never really threatened physical violence, on more than one occasion he'd slapped the wind out of me with his swift and stinging sarcasm.

Mr. Bunyan's apartment certainly wasn't the largest to be had in our retirement community, but I imagine it was the largest he could afford, and he was proud of it. The living room was good-sized, but, unfortunately, it appeared rather cramped, like the way a fresh new apartment always does when too much dark, heavy furniture from the former home is forced upon it.

By far, the best feature of the apartment was the balcony beyond the sliding glass doors, with its view of downtown Baltimore and the Inner Harbor. On a clear day, one could see the distant Francis Scott Key Bridge glimmering over the bay. Mr. Bunyan was particularly proud of that view. Sometimes, in the midst of arguing with me, he'd suddenly change the subject to that view, sweeping his big hand toward the sliding glass doors like he was lord of it all: open air, lots of it, carrying the weather over the roofs and treetops of the city—a silvering of snow, the sweet clarity of spring, the oppressive heat that Baltimore is famous for in the dog days of summer.

And then, of course, he'd return to the arguing.

Mostly we'd argue about whether Mr. Bunyan was really in trouble, alone in that apartment. I saw trouble aplenty: he was weak and getting weaker; he was vulnerable to falls, noncompliant with his diet and medications, and embarrassingly remiss in his personal hygiene. I was tactful, of course, in making my case.

Mr. Bunyan's opposing view was that he could manage just fine, if only I were more efficient in providing nursing assistants who could "get the job done"—bathing and personal care, housekeeping, laundry, meal preparation, medication management—in the few hours a week he'd allow them in. Mr. Bunyan was not particularly tactful in making his case. He referred to my staff as *your people,* as in "Your people never arrive on time" or "Your people have got my pill boxes all mixed up" or "Listen here, lady—tell your people that the food in my refrigerator belongs to me and I'll throw things out when I'm damned ready."

A more experienced and confident nurse would have quit arguing sooner. But I had just returned to nursing after years away. A divorce had borne down on me like my own personal tornado, leaving me bereft of purpose in my life. I coped by pinning my RN badge to my freshly ironed uniform jacket and striding out on rounds in my sensible new shoes. To each of my elderly charges I'd bring sunshine and sympathy and hope that things would turn out all right, if for no other reason than my appearance in their apartments. I was their good nurse, their true advocate.

Of course, it was vital to me that the residents liked me. Just about all of them did. All but Mr. Bunyan.

He would have none of my advocating for good nursing care. Instead, Mr. Bunyan made me his adversary.

A more experienced and confident nurse would have quit the arguing simply because of the obvious: inevitably, Mr. Bunyan would be wheeled out of the apartment in full-blown heart failure or suffering from either a fractured hip or a fractured skull, in which case neither of us could be declared the winner. My fear, of course, was that one day I'd knock and hear no irritated bark of reply, that I'd have to let myself in to find he'd died, alone, but sitting right where he wanted to be: in his recliner, the TV tray before him with its mess of half-eaten food and pill boxes, that stunning view of Baltimore behind him. No doubt Mr. Bunyan would have counted that one a win.

In the end, Mr. Bunyan did move to the health care center. As irony would have it, he moved when I was off for a few days, and so we both were spared the awkwardness of facing each other at such a sorry time. But remarkably—or perhaps this is the rare instance when "miraculously" applies—this story really ends some time earlier, on the day Mr. Bunyan and I achieved our truce.

It was a summer day, hot and humid outside, but unnaturally cold indoors with the air-conditioning blasting like a nor'easter. I could have used a sweater as I made my rounds, and it made me feel peevish that I felt so chilled all through the chaotic workday.

In my pocket I was carrying a list of nursing feats I could no longer imagine pulling off. In the back of my mind I was carrying heartache: the house in which I'd raised my children was up for sale and I was trapped in the letting go, unable to even step into the backyard where my cherished perennials—lilies and cosmos and black-eyed Susans—were now in bloom.

And so I knocked on Mr. Bunyan's door that day with my mind made up to take whatever blame he was prepared to heap on me, to bear up under the strain, to smile and back away—anything to get out of there without losing my grip.

As for Mr. Bunyan, he was having an inexplicably good day. He had only one complaint: that I kept sending him "new people," though he allowed that today's "little gal" seemed nice enough.

"Look at that beautiful day out there, will you, lady," he said, changing the subject, looking over his shoulder toward the view.

It wasn't a beautiful day. Beyond those sliding glass doors, the sky was gray with oppressive heat and haze, probably working itself up to a summer storm.

He frowned, studied my face. "Bad day?" he asked.

I pressed my lips into a smile. Suddenly, I couldn't speak, couldn't look him in the eye.

"You ought to step out there and take a breath of fresh air," he said. "It'll do you good. And while you're out there, why don't pick yourself one of my tomatoes."

I slid open the door and stepped into the heat of Mr. Bunyan's balcony.

He had moved his sickly houseplants out there, and someone had filled the window boxes with red geraniums. In the corner, leaning out through the railing, was a leggy tomato plant on which were ripening no more than a half-dozen tiny tomatoes.

He had said "one," so that was what I allowed myself: one small tomato, the size of a gumdrop. It was warm in my hand, firm. I held it carefully while I took in the view of the city. Thunder rumbled in the distance.

"Did you pick yourself a good ripe one?" Mr. Bunyan asked when I stepped inside.

I held it out for him to see—one small, ripe tomato, still warm from the sun, centered in my palm. "I'm going to save it," I said. "A treat for my lunch."

"You'll find it's sweet," he said. "Almost like dessert."

Afterward, going down the hall, I kept my hand in my pocket, still cradling that tomato. But later, alone in the elevator, I withdrew the tomato and placed it in my mouth. It was sweet indeed—a sort of communion, an offering of peace, hope that everything would be all right.

Acknowledgment of Permissions

"Breaking Bad News" is reprinted with the kind permission of Cortney Davis. The story was originally published in *MedHunters* magazine, Winter 2002, and online at www.medhuntersjournal.com.

"Cravings" is excerpted from *The Making of a Nurse* by Tilda Shalof © 2007. Published by McClelland & Stewart Ltd. Used with permission of the publisher.

"The Peaches" is reprinted with the kind permission of Nancy Leigh Harless. The story originally appeared in *Womankind: Connection and Wisdom Around the World*, released by Tate enterprises October 2007.

Reader's Guide

1. Dramatic events often spark hopeful times. Describe some of the events and patient cases that demonstrate hope in the stories you've read.

2. What are some ways to approach the challenge that Keynan Hobbs presents in "Julia," that of taking in another's suffering and letting it back out again? What resources do you have at your disposal to deal with this challenge? Does the idea of releasing the suffering seem superficial?

3. Dorothy Consonery-Fairnot reports about "Jim," a patient who never lost hope and never became depressed despite horrendous odds. In what ways can patients become sources of inspiration for nurses—and vice versa?

4. Doris Urfer and Karen Klein both write about nurses who changed their lives forever, compelling them both to become nurses. What was the

impetus behind your own career decision? Was there anyone specific who particularly inspired your choice? If so, who and in what way did that person affect your career path?

5. Think about your response to the question above regarding Doris Urfer's "My Life of Hope." Are there limits to what a nurse should do to offer support to her patient? How does the situation discussed in Mary Jeanne Creamer's "My Patient, My Hope" differ from the one in "My Life of Hope"? When is it appropriate to share personal information with a patient?

6. Tilda Shalof writes about the physical and emotional demands that nursing entails. How do these demands affect your spirit? The spirit of your patients? What can be done to protect your spirit?

7. Delivering bad or upsetting news is part of every nurse's job, as Cortney Davis wrote about in "Breaking Bad News." Have you ever had to receive bad news? What do you remember about that day? What does one look for when evaluating "the patient's emotional reserve"? What do you think about "soft peddling" bad news?

8. "Mr. Bunyan" gave Madeleine Mysko a rough time during his stay at her facility. Patients come with all sorts of issues and personalities. Think about a patient who has been especially difficult. How did you deal with that patient? Are there things you could have done differently?

9. A little lamp encapsulated and symbolized Bonnie Jarvis-Lowe's nursing career. This relic, from her nursing school days, held deep meaning for her. Think back to your days in nursing school. What gave you the hope and determination to carry on despite the tough times? Are there things or people—memories—that will help carry you through the good and the bad days during your career in healthcare?

10. Communication is at the heart of nursing: bonding with patients, discussing patient care with colleagues. Nancy Leigh Harless shares a story about how something lost in translation can actually bring people together by adding levity to a situation. How can humor and levity be used appropriately and successfully to help you navigate tricky situations with patients?

About the Editors

Paula Sergi, BSN, MFA, was selected by the Hessen Literary Society as the Wisconsin writer to act as the 2005 Cultural Ambassador for the Hessen-Wisconsin Writers Exchange. She is the author of *Family Business*, a collection of poems, and she co-edited *Boomer Girls: Poems by Women from the Baby Boom Generation*, University of Iowa Press, 1999. Sergi received a Wisconsin Arts Board Artist Fellowship in 2001. Her poetry is published regularly in such journals as *The Bellevue Literary Review, Primavera, Crab Orchard Review, and Spoon River Poetry Review* and her writing has been featured recently in the *American Journal of Nursing*. She worked as a staff nurse at University of Wisconsin Hospitals, as a public health nurse with various county departments, and as a visiting nurse in Portland, Oregon. Now she focuses her time as a teacher and writer. She teaches creative writing at Ripon College, and lives in Fond du Lac, Wisconsin.

Geraldine Gorman, RN, PhD, is an Assistant Professor in the College of Nursing at the University of Illinois at Chicago. She holds an M.A. in English Literature and a PhD in Nursing, both from Loyola University, Chicago. Before coming to UIC in 2002, she taught at Western Michigan University. Prior to entering the nursing profession in 1991, she taught writing as a teaching assistant at Loyola University. She also worked in direct social services, living in community at the Little Brothers of the Poor and participating in all aspects of their service to low-income elderly, including meal delivery, relocation services, and holiday and vacation celebrations. In this capacity, she also facilitated poetry workshops in nursing homes, resulting in two small anthologies of collected work. She was a founding member of a small grass roots organization in Tempe, AZ, which served the needs of the many relocated elderly and she organized the local university community to provide, among other services, respite care for the spouses of Alzheimer victims. Before beginning nursing school, Gerry served as the volunteer coordinator and editorial assistant to H.O.M.E, a nonprofit housing organization for Chicago's low-income elderly.

About the Contributors

Dorothy Consonery-Fairnot, MSHA, RN, CCM, CLNC, is southeast regional manager over field case management for MedInsights. She manages nurses in ten states who provide medical case management and rehabilitative services to assist injured workers in receiving the appropriate medical care. Ms. Consonery-Fairnot has more than thirty-five years of diversified nursing experience and holds a master's degree in health care services administration. She also is a certified case manager and legal nurse consultant. Ms. Consonery-Fairnot has been published in several professional journals including *Lippincott's Case Management, Care Management, CARING, The Health Care Executive*, and *The Rehab Pro*. She is a member of the board of directors for the Commission for Case Management Certification.

Mary Jeanne Creamer, BSN, graduated from SUNY Farmingdale with an associate's degree and earned her BSN from SUNY Stonybrook. She currently is enrolled in a master's program and recently obtained a position as a nursing instructor.

Cortney Davis, MA, RNC, APRN, is a nurse practitioner in women's health, is the author of *I Knew a Woman* (Random House), which won the Center for the Book's 2002 award for nonfiction. Davis's poetry collections include *The Body Flute* and *Details of Flesh*. Her most recent collection, *Leopold's Maneuvers* (University of Nebraska Press), won the 2003 Prairie Schooner Book Prize. Coeditor of two anthologies of poetry and prose by nurses, *Between the Heartbeats and Intensive Care* (University of Iowa Press), Davis has been awarded an NEA Poetry Fellowship and two Connecticut Commission Poetry Grants.

Jessica Gallinaro, RN, currently works at New York Presbyterian Hospital/Weill Cornell Medical center as the Patient Care Director of a cardiac stepdown unit. She is from Long Island, graduated from Georgetown University in 2004, and has been living and working in New York City ever since.

Amanda Goodwin is currently completing her BSN-RN at Kent State University. Driven by a compassion only a personal history of chronic illness could provide, Amanda is excited to begin a career in pediatric critical care nursing. Amanda is passionate about life and especially enjoys traveling and scrapbooking.

Patricia Harman, **RN, CNM, MSN**, is a nurse-midwife in private practice in Morgantown, West Virginia, and the author of *The Blue Cotton Gown: A Midwife's Memoir* (Beacon, 2008). She is an assistant clinical professor on the faculty of the school of medicine and the school of nursing at West Virginia University.

Nancy Leigh Harless's stories have been included in many anthologies including *Cup of Comfort, The Healing Project, Chicken Soup for the Soul,* and *Travelers Tales,* as well as many professional and literary journals. A graduate of Intercollegiate Center for Nursing Education in Spokane, Washington, she worked largely in the area of Maternal Child Health before receiving her advanced degree, as a Women's Healthcare Nurse Practitioner.

Keynan Hobbs, **MSN, RN**, is a psychiatric/mental health clinical nurse specialist at an inner-city hospital in San Diego, California. He trained for advanced practice in psychiatric nursing at the Philadelphia Veterans Administration Medical Center while attending the University of Pennsylvania.

Patricia Holloran, RN, has worked in many areas of nursing for the past 35 years, with the last eight years in substance abuse. She has been very active in helping to obtain an alternative to discipline program for health professionals that are impaired by substance abuse, or mental illness in her state of CT. She is the author of *Impaired: A Nurse's Story of Addiction and Recovery.*

Karen Klein, **RN**, is a magna cum laude graduate with a Bachelor of Science in Nursing from Adelphi University. Her varied nursing experience includes ER/Trauma, Pediatrics, Interventional Radiology, Telemetry, ICU, Home Infusion, and Occupational Health. She is a Certified Emergency Nurse and an AHA CPR/First Aid Instructor, and has been published by *Nursing Spectrum Magazine.*

Bonnie Jarvis-Lowe, RN, is a trained nurse, graduating from the Grace General Hospital School of Nursing in 1969. Now retired, she spent most of her nursing career in Nova Scotia. She began her career in nursing in the operating room and then switched to bedside nursing after seventeen years.

Emily J. McGee, RN, MSN, APRN-BC, NREMT-P, is a flight nurse at Aero Med in Grand Rapids, Michigan. She is also a nurse and captain in the U.S. Army

Reserves, and works as an emergency room nurse practitioner. In her spare time, McGee writes about flight nursing at *www.crzegrl.net*. Her hobbies include anything involving massive amounts of adrenaline.

Rashida J. Merchant, BScN, RN, RM, has been associated with the Aga Khan University Hospital (AKUH) in Karachi, Pakistan, since 1986. After completing her studies in general nursing and midwifery in 1986, she started as a bedside nurse and has served as a manager of Maternal and Child Care Areas, Nursing Education Services, and Nursing Recruitment Office. She completed her Post-RN BScN work, with honors, in 1999. Ms. Merchant is an active member of Treasurer of Rho Delta Chapter, Sigma Theta Tau International, is a facilitator tool trainer for Quality Circles, and is a trained facilitator for continuous quality improvement activities.

Laura Monahan has worked as a construction welder (welding oil tanks and pressure vessels) and a power plant operator at an electrical utility, while attending college, where she graduated with highest honors. She attained a MBA at Northwestern's Kellogg Graduate School of Management (graduated top quarter), while working various management positions, the last one negotiating long-term power contracts between utilities in the United States and Canada. She then quit working to raise her second child. During that time, she started a mural business, and built her own house. Now, she is in nursing school pursuing another dream and having lots of fun.

Madeleine Mysko's work, both poetry and prose, has been published in such venues as *The Hudson Review, Shenandoah, Commonweal, River Styx, The Christian Century*, and *The Baltimore Sun*. A graduate of The Writing Seminars of The Johns Hopkins University, she teaches creative writing both privately and in the Johns Hopkins Advanced Academic Programs. She is also a registered nurse with experience in Assisted Living. Among her awards are two Individual Artist grants from the Maryland State Arts Council, a Howard Nemerov Sonnet Award, and an Artscape Prize for Fiction from the City of Baltimore.

Mary H. Palmer, PhD, RNC, FAAN, was raised in Baltimore, Maryland, and is a graduate of the University of Maryland at Baltimore School of Nursing. She was awarded her PhD in 1990 from Johns Hopkins University School of Hygiene and Public Health and her MFA from Goddard College in 1999. She is a Professor at The University of North Carolina at Chapel Hill School of Nursing.

Angela Posey-Arnold, RN, BSN, is a published Christian author and retired RN, living with her husband of 20 years in a log home in beautiful northwest Alabama. Her writing and music studio, Pebble East Studios, is located in the loft of the log home. Ms. Posey-Arnold has been widely published, with two Christian nonfiction books, many short stories, Christian articles, devotionals, and poetry. Her work also has been featured in *Faith Writers Magazine* and she is a regular contributing writer for the popular e-zine *www.4Him2U.com*. Her newest book is *The Nightingale Protocol*.

Barbara Gordon Sauvage, an RN who has worked in Emergency Medicine as well as Hospice, is in the last throes of her Master's in Nursing at University of Illinois—Chicago. She is married, and has two grown daughters, neither of whom are named Skipper.

Tilda Shalof, RN, BScN, is an intensive care unit nurse with twenty years of experience in Israel, New York, and Canada. Her first book, *A Nurse's Story: Life, Death, and In-Between in an Intensive Care Unit*, was a bestseller that received rave reviews.

Elizabeth Tibbetts's book of poems *In the Well* (2003) won the Bluestem Poetry Award. Her work appears in journals such as The American Scholar, Prairie Schooner, and Spoon River Poetry Review, and has been featured on The Writer's Almanac. She works as a registered nurse in an acute care setting.

Doris I. Urfer, LPN, was born in Las Martinas, Cuba. Seventeen years later, she was forced to leave the country with her family and moved to the United States. She worked as a key punch operator for many years until her daughter inspired her to go into nursing school. Doris has been an LPN for twenty-five years and is near retirement.

Eileen Valinoti, RN, is a registered nurse. Her essays have appeared in *Glamour, Parents*, and *Health* magazines and in nursing journals. In 2007 her short story "Night Duty" was published in *The Healing Muse*, a literary magazine.

K. Lynn Wieck, PhD, RN, is CEO of Management Solutions for Healthcare and is a nurse consultant for health policy and workforce issues. She is also the Jacqueline M. Braithwaite Professor at the University of Texas at Tyler. Dr. Wieck has published six nursing textbooks which have been translated into five languages and wrote a monthly column about nursing for the *Houston Chronicle* for four years. Her latest book,

Stories for Nurses: Acts of Caring was released in August 2002 and received an *American Journal of Nursing* Book of the Year award.

Reflections on Doctors

Nurses' Stories about Physicians and Surgeons

~

Terry Ratner, RN, MFA
EDITOR

Home Delivery

~

Cara Muhlhahn, CNM

I LOVE MY WORK, love every one of my patients, love being in private practice. I derive incredible satisfaction as a home-birth midwife from helping women become mothers in the most natural, safe, and empowered way. But there are many uphill battles in this field, especially these days, when home-birth midwives still need to fight for legitimacy. Things are gradually changing for the better, but there are still so many misperceptions about who we are and what we do.

A compliment I received from one father says it all. He was fine with the idea of home birth from the beginning. But the baby came out not breathing and I had to do a neonatal resuscitation. It was the Fourth of July. The dad had called 911, at my request, just in case the resuscitation was not a success—which it was. At the end, when I was cleaning up the birthing pool, he came up to me and complimented me on how well I'd done, and on my "professional comportment."

He was incredibly relieved that I could successfully perform a resuscitation when needed. I don't think he ever considered that it might be possible. At the time I thought, "What did he expect?" But in hindsight I understand that patients and their partners don't necessarily understand that we're medically trained birthing professionals.

Before meeting me, this new dad had probably expected me to be some touchy-feely, matronly hippie equipped to offer little more than moral support, a hand to hold, and maybe some arcane, esoteric "wisewoman's" wisdom—all of which is probably quite helpful. He didn't expect me to be the serious, capable clinician that I am. I'm sure that his image of a midwife was forever changed.

It's not just the general public who's confused, but doctors as well. And the fact that there are so many routes of entry into midwifery creates even more confusion within the field. There are CNMs (certified nurse midwives), like me; CMs (certified midwives); and CPMs (certified professional midwives). The various groups of midwives have different levels of education and are standardized and regulated by different bodies that often disagree about things like protocols for licensure. And then there are midwives who have come to the profession through an unregulated apprenticeship. This confusion makes it more difficult to win political gains and the trust of the women who are thinking about choosing midwives.

Among the most frustrating of our hurdles is American doctors' misconceptions, because the medical field and its governing bodies—the American College of Obstetrics and Gynecology (ACOG), for example—have such influence over public opinion. In February 2008, ACOG released a statement reiterating their opposition to home birth—rather ignorantly, especially when considering that 70 percent of births in Europe and Japan are done at home.

DESPITE THE MISCONCEPTIONS, there are still physicians who manage to support women making empowering choices. Some doctors have taken the time to understand what home birth is about and what midwives do, and they are very supportive of us and our patients. I have been fortunate to find some with whom I can work, and I am grateful for them and all their referrals to my practice. I work regularly with a perinatologist, a cardiologist, a hematologist, holistic gynecologist, assorted ob-gyns, pediatricians, and psychologists. When we work in tandem, supporting one another, great things can happen.

And hospitals aren't all bad. We couldn't do without them in cases of emergency. They have intelligent doctors, machines, high-tech equipment, and medications on hand that are great to have access to when things are abnormal or dangerous. They're just not great places for normal birth.

Here's an example of a great collaboration between a couple of doctors and a midwife, and ways in which a hospital can even be helpful in supporting home birth. Sabine, a German-born patient of mine, had her first baby with Dr. Jacques Moritz, an ob-gyn colleague. Everything went fine. Dr. Moritz sent her my way when he knew that she was seeking a home birth for her second child.

Sabine's second pregnancy went beautifully. The baby grew normally in the third trimester. At the 32-week point, the head should begin to present, and the doctor or midwife checks to see that it's doing so. Sabine's baby's head was in a position that we call *oblique*, which means that instead of being directly in the pelvis, right over the pubic bone, it was a bit off to the side.

Toward the end of a woman's pregnancy, the prenatal visits get closer. Each time I came to see Sabine, I saw that her baby's head was moving slowly from oblique to transverse. At each visit I gently coaxed it back into the center, without duress, checking in on the baby's heartbeat to see if it minded, and it didn't.

From about the 37th week of a woman's pregnancy until delivery, I see her even more frequently—about once a week. During that time with Sabine, I noticed that the baby's head was moving slowly up toward the fundus, the top of the uterus. It seemed the baby was sneaking into a breech presentation. This was especially interesting to me because it recalled what my mother had told me about my time in utero: how the doctor kept turning me, but by the time we'd return for the next visit, I would revert to breech position.

I knew there had to be a reason this baby was turning the way it was. So I decided to take Sabine in for a sonogram to see where the cord was. I had a sneaking suspicion that the cord was around the neck, which is not usually a problem and occurs in 40 percent of normal deliveries. In this case, however, I thought it might be responsible for the baby's continuous journey northward.

Sabine and I went together to my perinatologist, Dr. Franz Margono at Saint Vincent's Hospital. We notified her husband, Ronnie, about what was going on and he went to meet us there. Dr. Margono did the sonogram and determined that the cord was twice around the neck and gave us advice to not "*schwinger*" the baby, using the German word for "swing," although it sounded more like *schvingeh*.

We explored the underlying meaning of Dr. Margono's advice for the next two hours or so at dinner nearby, where Ronnie joined us. I explained the situation to them, and laid out all the options. The implication of what Dr. Margono said was that I shouldn't force the baby back into a vertex presentation. *Ay, ay, ay,* I thought. If we couldn't get the baby back into a vertex presentation, then our options were quickly narrowing to a cesarean section, at least as our perinatologist saw it. I had a feeling, though, that things weren't so bleak. My instincts told me there was a way for Sabine to fulfill her dream of a home birth—or at the very least a vaginal birth rather than a C-section.

So I came up with a plan. Up until our last visit, I had been gently urging the baby from oblique and transverse to vertex without a problem as evidenced by my Doppler fetal heart rate. Of course, I was wrestling with the part of me that saw fit to bring Sabine in for a sonogram in the first place because the head was continuously rising in her uterus. I phoned Dr. Moritz, Sabine's former obstetrician, and asked him if he could turn the baby in the hospital as a way of ensuring that the baby tolerated the turning. There we would be able to monitor the baby after the turning. This might mean that Sabine would be induced to get her labor started before the baby could turn back around. Then, we'd head back to their place for a home birth.

For her part, Sabine would have been happy if I had just turned her baby once more. But I felt cautious with this new information about the cord wrapped twice around the baby's neck, and felt the heat of Dr. Margono's wagging "*no schvingeh*" finger. At this point, I was reluctant to turn the baby. My gut was telling me not to and I felt compelled to listen to it. I was still optimistic about the chances for a home birth, although Ronnie finally confessed to Sabine that "I was happy to go along with the home birth as long as things remained low-risk, but things have changed."

Dr. Moritz agreed to my plan. But the day Sabine went in ended up being extremely busy at the hospital, an inadvertent blessing in disguise. Sabine and Ronnie were there all day. After a long wait, the baby was easily turned. The doctor who did the turning said that it was possible that the cord was actually just laying over the shoulder, not wrapped around the neck twice as it had appeared to Dr. Margono. He explained that sonography is not a perfect science.

Many hours after turning, the baby was monitored and doing fine. Dr. Moritz was supposed to stop by, but his office hours were keeping him. In the meantime, Ronnie called me to say that the doctor who turned the baby was pushing for a hospital delivery.

The doctor told him, "Hey, you've played with this baby enough. Let's just get him out." This made Ronnie really anxious. He didn't want to do anything that would put the baby at risk.

I asked Ronnie if he—a professor—thought that the doctor had presented him with a well-thought-out risk-benefit analysis of the situation that made sense to him, as I had done the other night at dinner.

"No," he allowed. But he was uncertain how to proceed—due, of course, to the weight the doctor's statement carried.

I said to Ronnie, "Maybe this doctor is just opposed to home birth." When pressed by Ronnie, he revealed his bias against it.

Sabine had no problem sticking to her guns in the face of all of these medical assessments. Ronnie was doing his best to conquer his own fears, which were being exploited by the doctor who'd turned the baby. I finally got Dr. Moritz on the phone while they were at the hospital, and we talked. He said the baby had been monitored there all day and was doing fine.

I asked him, "If Sabine and Ronnie want to go ahead with the home birth, would you take us back in the hospital in the event that the baby experienced any distress?" The reason this had to be negotiated at that point was because I didn't feel comfortable, in the event of transfer, bringing Sabine back to Saint Vincent's having *schvinged*, albeit in the hospital under surveillance for the whole day.

Dr. Moritz said, "Sure." My kind of doctor.

Ronnie and Sabine came across town to my office. We made a plan for induction that night so the baby wouldn't have a chance to turn back around. The induction plan involved administration of castor oil. I decided to sleep at their house, Doppler-armed so as to make everyone—including myself—comfortable with the baby's status.

I listened to the baby all night. The signs were all good. The castor oil kicked in gradually and the labor proceeded slowly during the course of the day, as some second labors do. Sabine's doula was there. Things just didn't seem to be moving and so we all made a plan to go take a walk on the roof of their building. As soon as we were there for about 15 minutes, I had to guide everyone back down again, as Sabine's contractions became strong and steady. We went inside and I got things ready for the birth. Within half an hour her water broke and the baby came out.

And guess what! Dr. Margono was right. The cord was around the neck twice, but not tightly at all. If it had been tight, I could have handled it by cutting it, but I didn't need to in this case. I just gently lifted the cord over the baby's head once, then again, and he came out and breathed...well, beautifully. Sabine was on top of the world. She did it! I was thrilled, to say the least. And Ronnie was too.

By taking things one step at a time, unhurriedly, and by incorporating all of the parents' feelings—as well as those of the experts—we reached a great conclusion. *Yay!* One more unnecessary cesarean avoided because of excellent clinical management and great collaboration with doctors.

Nurse Cherry Ames and Dr. Fortune Marry

~

Paula Sergi, RN, MFA

I USUALLY WAIT UNTIL I know someone quite well before revealing that I am married to a doctor. My reluctance to discuss my husband's profession is multifaceted and includes a Midwestern sensibility of modesty.

There's also the fact that I've lived through the second wave of feminism and like to believe that my own work is of greater interest than my husband's profession. I imagine that there was a time when the opposite was true; that women would readily announce their Mrs. Doctor status, savoring the prestige it afforded them.

Maybe it's because I'm a nurse and am biased, but these days I perceive a growing distrust and even disdain for the medical profession. The mere mention of the word *physician* brings up images of headstrong, bossy, egocentric people who have little respect for their coworkers. I know because I worked as a student nurse and staff nurse long before meeting my husband.

His career choice would have worked against him at the beginning of our courtship had his intelligence, warmth, ability to cook, and love of the arts not been immediately obvious. So it's hurtful to me to listen to grumbling and doctor-bashing; that is, unless the conversation addresses all aspects of healthcare reform.

There are quirky conditions that surround the doctor-nurse marriage. The most obvious is the quick mental leap to the stereotypical relationship made famous by novels from the 1940s and 1950s. Old concepts linger, and they are not flattering to anyone. Book covers featured a doctor looking lecherously at a pretty blond nurse. Remember Nurse Cherry Ames and Dr. Joseph Fortune? Despite her dedication and cleverness, she seemed to always be under his influence. The literature informing contemporary culture has promoted the notion that the most a nurse can hope for is to be the object of a male physician's lust. This bit of fiction masks the rich give-and-take that characterizes relationships between nurses and physicians, at work and at home.

Other ramifications are equally infuriating, like the situation I encountered one day when I was late for my son's sporting event and took a seat next to another mother. "I was working the immunization clinic," I explained.

"What do you do there?" she asked.

"I give the shots."

"Did your husband teach you to do that?" she wondered aloud.

Never mind my BS degree or ten years as a public-health nurse. The idea that just being married to a physician would allow me to be on the payroll of the local public health department infuriated me, despite my understanding that naiveté and ignorance were at the heart of that woman's comment.

Such ignorance is not wholly uncommon. We live in a small community and there's a weird curiosity about doctors' lives that hovers ominously. Though 40,000 people is not quite Andy Griffith's Mayberry, we have a large population at and above retirement age. Some really do listen to the police scanner as a hobby. When my husband was hospitalized for a kidney stone, the rumors included that he had suffered a heart attack brought on by my having left him. The convoluted facts about my husband's medical condition and the state of our marriage apparently were delicious to the hospital employees.

A weaker marriage would not survive the stresses that my husband's work has brought to our family. The number of meals we've had together in the last 23 years is minimal, because after a full day of hospital and clinic work, he returns calls to his patients and dictates his notes from the day. He also makes house calls to patients who are too ill to leave home or who are in the last stages of their lives. He attends his patients' funerals as a last gesture of care and respect.

People assume that the financial rewards compensate for evenings, weekends, holidays, and birthdays spent without my husband. The idea of being a physician's wife or child conjures piles of money at our disposal for all kinds of uses, and privileges galore. I know because I grew up poor and heard my neighbors, relatives, and the general public express these ideas in casual conversation and discourse.

Our children grew up knowing that their father's work took precedence, that he would be away long hours, and that bedtime stories, their sporting events, and elementary school performances were no exception. For a while, I worried about how this would affect them, but I was always aware of my husband's special warmth and of his ability to communicate his love and concern to our children. When I ask my now-young-

adult sons about this they claim to have no resent-
ment at all. "I always understood the importance of
his work," they say, "and how he was helping people."
They indicate that they might have resented his time
away if he'd been on the golf course or playing cards
or at a bar. But they knew he was always with sick
people, and that was understandable to them.

My husband is not a saint. He has high expectations for himself and for those around him and these
expectations sometimes are relayed in a shorthand
that can be interpreted as critical. I have heard him
ask a nurse to straighten the notepad messages in a
patient chart because it is a legal document, and as
such should not appear sloppy. This kind of attention
to detail is not without merit but can be difficult to
address when so many other tasks are pressing in a
nurse's day.

As he ages, his perspective is becoming more
rigid. He cannot understand his younger colleagues,
whose primary concerns seem to be time off and sal-
ary. He is frustrated with the difficulties in attract-
ing and keeping younger physicians in the internal
medicine practice in which he is a partner. He has
become intolerant of colleagues who do not hold or
demonstrate good patient care as the gold standard by
which they act and with administrators who haven't
yet considered it, despite their lingo. He is tired of

being called to wipe up the messes that surgeons leave behind. He is sad that his profession is all but lost, and blames physicians themselves for this sorry state.

Being married to a person who is totally committed to his work has its shortcomings. But it also demonstrates to our children the values of compassion, of a commitment to having high standards. It gives us a lot to be proud of. I don't have to mention this when I meet someone for the first time. Let them wonder about the person behind the woman who attends social functions alone and is not afraid to set the record straight about life as a nurse married to a doctor.

A Truth about Cats
and Dogs

~

Adrienne Zurub, RN, MA, CNOR

Mornings are not supposed to smell like burning flesh with wispy twirls of flesh smoke moving sensually and methodically toward the cluster of operating-room lights. Morning sounds should not be muffled weeping or verbalized grimaces. The sounds of morning should not allow the normalcy of the electric saw making its way through the guardian bone of sternum, thus literally exposing someone's heart to the world. Yet for me these were my mornings for more than 25 years.

This setting, barbaric in any sense of the word, was the backdrop of my experience as a cardiothoracic surgical RN (formerly) on the open heart-heart transplant team at Cleveland Clinic. These ORs were my battleground and playground. Those experiences and visuals, and their accompanying sensations—good and bad—became the foreground of my holistic collage.

The fugitive truth is that those sounds, that weeping and those grimaces by patients (and staff alike) become talismans that we (nurses and surgeons) carry the rest of our respective lives. Often, I viewed the surgeons I worked with as automatons in the OR. And indeed some surgeons acquire this "distancing" veneer in order to do the necessary work.

In our cardiothoracic operating rooms, an over-arching competitive environment exists. Arrogance, entitlement, outstanding talents (nurses and surgeons), and palpable confidence dominate the entire operating-room suites. A nurse pushes herself or himself through this encompassing fog of testosterone. I say *testosterone* because the surgeons, the ones who are in charge, are all male. To work in this environment, one has to have the personality and the chutzpah—the balls—to think quickly and react perfectly. Weakness or hesitation is normally not considered an option.

So it was with great surprise that I was approached one late evening, as I sat at the cardiac control desk, by a new staff surgeon who had lost a patient. During the exchange, I came to realize how remarkable the distancing has to be in order for this new staff guy to do his job and perform extraordinary feats of surgery. I also realized in those moments that I was the one who resided in a protective callus acquired from years of experience, years of death, and the pain of knowing. My sense of efficacy allowed that this OR death and its cognitive talisman would be one of many that he (like me) will carry the rest of our lives in our efforts to help others.

In this one illuminating moment, the distance and power dynamic between the two forces, that of nurse and doctor, are somehow bridged. Here we are one. The hospital-induced power differential is turned on its head, as I, being the experienced nurse, am deemed the wise one, the resource, and a confidante. There was simply in our communication the active current of humanness that permeated the space between us.

He stood before me, crushed and battered at his first operating-room death. He wept openly before me, making me uncomfortable. I am accustomed to fits of rage, screaming, yelling, sulkiness, and a bit of (okay, a lot of) berating for the failure, the mistake, and falling short of expectations and the realization that they (heart surgeons) too are simply human.

He may realize that no matter what surgical algorithm he performs on patients that present to him, some patients will rightfully die. This is not an indictment, or an acquiescence of hope, but simply the reality of man versus destiny or a divine force.

This OR beckons to those patients who have no place else to go. Those who have been told by the second and third opinion to "go home and comfortably die." We are the last hope for these extremely high-acuity patients...and sometimes their last stop. Although many of the patients know this upon entering our OR, their families do not always understand.

Years ago, the surgeons appeared to love the thrill of the cases that were deemed impossible and time-consuming. Those guys were machinelike, churning out successes and making history. The newer guys are more...human. They desire success, but not at the expense of their family and a life.

So, I am heartened by this surgeon's 21st-century attitude. It is an attitude that, at least for now, shows that he does not need to step on me or my fellow colleagues. He is young and not yet institutionalized to the vagaries of our power hierarchy. Now he is willing to show his vulnerability.

I wonder what this new surgeon's—the one with the size-eight hands—reaction will be in, say, ten years or even a year from now. I wonder if this loss will be his "Moby Dick" in the continual pursuit and war against heart disease. Which patients will stay with him and further hone his skills with their respective challenges? Which patients will leave the remnants of themselves forever on his psyche...as they have left the talismans of themselves on me? Right now, he and I are partners.

Share Your Stories
with Kaplan Publishing

KAPLAN PUBLISHING, THE #1 educational resource for nurses, would like to feature your story in an upcoming anthology in the *Kaplan Voices: Nurses* series. Please share the stories behind the relationships, experiences, and issues you encounter on the job—whether you work in a hospital, clinic, home setting, hospice, private medical practice, or elsewhere.

Entertaining and educational, inspirational and practical, each *Kaplan Voices: Nurses* anthology features true stories written by nurses about the experiences and relationships that inspire and enrich their lives and all those who come into contact with them.

FOR WRITER'S GUIDELINES or to join our mailing list, please contact Kaplan Publishing by email at *kaplanvoicesnurses@gmail.com*, or write to us at:

Nurse Stories
Editorial Assistant
Kaplan Publishing
1 Liberty Plaza, 24th Floor
New York, NY 10006, USA

More Nursing Books
Available From Kaplan

Notes on Nursing
    Florence Nightingale
    978-1-4277-9797-1 $9.95

Your Career in Nursing, 5th Edition
    Annette Vallano, MS, RN, APRN, BC
    978-1-4277-9787-2 $17.00

First Year Nurse
    Barbara Arnoldussen, RN, MBA
    978-1-4195-5116-1 $12.00

How to Survive Clinical
    Diann L. Martin, PhD, RN
    978-1-4277-9822-0 $12.95

Labor of Love: A Midwife's Memoir
    Cara Muhlhahn, CNM
    978-1-4277-9821-3 $25.95   (available January 2009)

Saving Lives: Why the Media's Portrayal
of Nurses Puts Healthcare at Risk
    Sandy Summers, MSN, MPH, RN
    Harry Jacob Summers, JD
    978-1-4277-9845-9 $24.95   (available January 2009)

AVAILABLE WHEREVER BOOKS ARE SOLD!